Learning Cardiac Magnetic Resonance

Massimo Imazio • Monica Andriani
Luisa Lobetti Bodoni • Fiorenzo Gaita

Learning Cardiac Magnetic Resonance

A Case-Based Guide

Springer

Massimo Imazio
Cardiovascular and Thoracic Department
AOU Città della Salute e della Scienza di Torino, University Cardiology
Turin
Italy

Monica Andriani
Cardiovascular and Thoracic Department
AOU Città della Salute e della Scienza di Torino, University Cardiology
Turin
Italy

Luisa Lobetti Bodoni
Radiology Department
AOU Città della Salute e della Scienza di Torino
Turin
Italy

Fiorenzo Gaita
Department of Medical Science
University of Turin
Turin
Italy

ISBN 978-3-030-11607-1 ISBN 978-3-030-11608-8 (eBook)
https://doi.org/10.1007/978-3-030-11608-8

This Springer imprint is published by the registered company Springer Nature Switzerland AG
The registered company address is: Gewerbestrasse 11, 6330 Cham, Switzerland

Foreword

Cardiac magnetic resonance (CMR) is the gold standard for the evaluation of biventricular volumes and function and has the unique capability (among other imaging techniques) to provide a good non-invasive tissue characterization (e.g. detection of oedema, fibro-fatty replacement, and scars). The number of these exams is increasing year by year and a basic knowledge of the indications, contraindications and advantages of CMR is essential for cardiologists, and especially new cardiologists in training, since this technique will become more and more essential and integrated with other imaging modalities in the future. There are so many books in English dealing with CMR. Why a new one? Most books do not provide a concise basic overview of the technique for non-experts. This book is an essential introduction to the study of CMR to allow a first orientation and provide an easy-to-read text for those who are interested to learn CMR or have started learning CMR. In addition, the book can be useful for clinicians (not experts in CMR), who simply want to understand the basics of CMR, its diagnostic capabilities and limitations compared with other imaging techniques, especially echocardiography. The book has been written by cardiologists and radiologists, who also work together in order to provide the best analysis and reporting for patients in clinical practice.

Professor Mauro Rinaldi
Director of the Cardiovascular and Thoracic Department
AOU Città della Salute e della Scienza di Torino
Turin, Italy

Contents

Contributors

Monica Andriani Cardiovascular and Thoracic Department, AOU Città della Salute e della Scienza di Torino, University Cardiology, Turin, Italy

Luisa Lobetti Bodoni Radiology Department, AOU Città della Salute e della Scienza di Torino, Turin, Italy

Fiorenzo Gaita Department of Medical Science, University of Turin, Turin, Italy

Massimo Imazio Cardiovascular and Thoracic Department, AOU Città della Salute e della Scienza di Torino, University Cardiology, Turin, Italy

Basic Physics for Clinicians

1

Contents

1.1 Introduction and Clinical Indications

Cardiac magnetic resonance (CMR) is becoming an increasingly popular imaging diagnostic modality being able to answer to a number of different questions in many cardiovascular diseases with the unique capability to provide a comprehensive assessment of the cardiovascular system without using ionizing radiation. The aim

M. Imazio et al., *Learning Cardiac Magnetic Resonance*,
https://doi.org/10.1007/978-3-030-11608-8_1

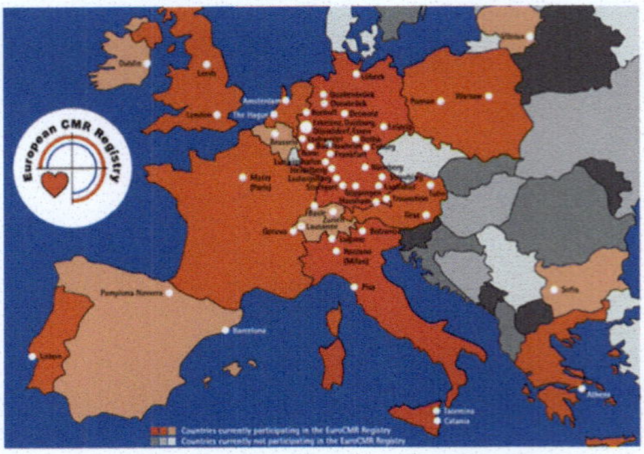

EuroCMR registry

	≤44 yrs	45 – 59 yrs	60 – 74 yrs	≥75 yrs
Indication				
Ischemia/CAD	12.1%	37.7%	48.1%	49.5%
Myocarditis/CMP	63.6%	36.6%	22.5%	16.5%
Viability	5.3%	17.0%	19.2%	22.4%
Stress CMR	13.7%	38.0%	47.5%	47.9%

Fig. 1.1 The EuroCMR registry and most common indications for cardiac MR according to this registry

Table 1.1 Common indications for cardiac magnetic resonance (CMR)

1. Suspected myocarditis
2. Heart failure and cardiomyopathies
3. Ischemia detection (vasodilator stress perfusion) and viability assessment
4. Congenital heart diseases and abnormal course of coronary arteries
5. Diseases of the aorta
6. Cardiac masses
7. Pericardial diseases
8. Heart valve diseases

of the present chapter is to provide an overview of the key physical principles of CMR for clinicians [1–6].

According to the EuroCMR registry [1], a multicentre registry with consecutive enrolment of more than 27,000 patients in 57 centres in 15 European countries, the most important indications were risk stratification in suspected CAD/ischemia (34.2%), workup of myocarditis/cardiomyopathies (32.2%) as well as assessment of viability (14.6%) (Fig. 1.1).

CMR provided diagnostic image quality in more than 98% without mortality and with severe complications in less than 0.1%, always associated with stress testing. Moreover CMR findings had an impact on patient management in more than 60% of cases with a new diagnosis in about 9% of cases [1].

Compared with echocardiography, CMR offers the opportunity to assess patients with poor acustic windows (e.g. patients with lung diseases, COPD) and to assess any part of the body regardless of its composition being able to improve our capability to characterize the nature of the tissue (e.g. watery content, fat, muscle, inflammation and fibrosis). This can occur without fixed imaging windows, such as in echocardiography, and irrespective of the body habitus [2].

Common indications for CMR study are listed in Table 1.1.

1.2 Basics of MR Physics

The basic of CMR is how the signal is generated. In CMR, the signal is generated by excitation of the hydrogen nuclei within free water or lipid molecules by radiofrequencies (RF). The hydrogen nucleus is a proton that acts as a little bore magnet (Fig. 1.2).

In the absence of a magnetic field, each hydrogen nucleus is randomly oriented (the net magnetic field is zero). When the hydrogen nuclei are put in a magnetic field as in the CMR scan, they align parallel (most of them) or antiparallel to the magnetic field. Since there is a slight excess of hydrogen nuclei oriented in the direction of the magnetic field, this creates a net magnetic field vector. This net magnetic vector is used to generate the CMR signal. The greater the applied magnetic field strength, Bo, the greater the excess of protons aligned with the magnetic field and the greater the size of the net magnetization (thus a 3.0 tesla magnet will generate a stronger signal than a 1.5 tesla magnet).

Each proton in the hydrogen nuclei does not simply line in the direction or against the direction of the magnetic field but also revolves (spin) on its axis: this phenomenon is called precession. The frequency of this precession is directly proportional to the magnetic field strength. The relation (Larmor equation) is

$$\text{Larmor frequency} = \text{Constant} \times \text{Bo}$$

The Larmor frequency is proportional to the strength of the magnetic field and is typically in the megahertz range, e.g. for 1.5 T, the Larmor frequency is 63 MHz. This is also known as the resonant frequency, since the protons only absorb energy

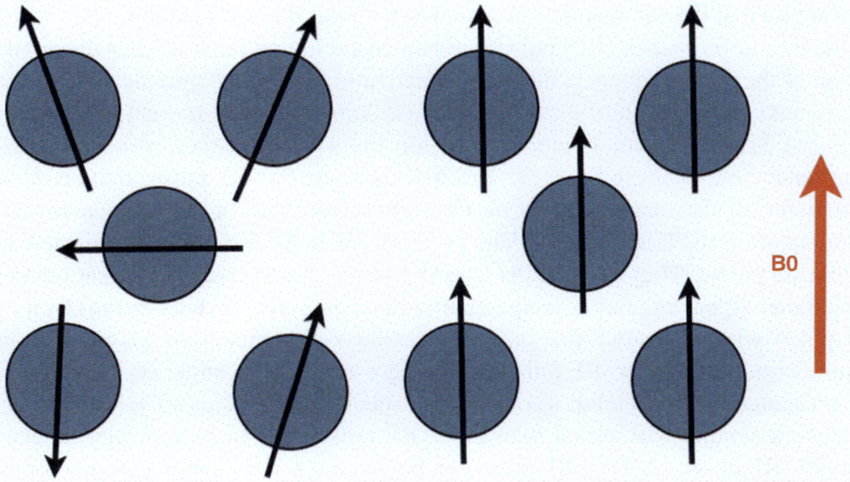

Fig. 1.2 The hydrogen nucleus is a proton that acts as a little bore magnet. In the absence of a magnetic field, each hydrogen nucleus is randomly oriented (the net magnetic field is zero). When the hydrogen nuclei are put in a magnetic field as in the CMR scan, they align parallel (most of them) or antiparallel to the magnetic field

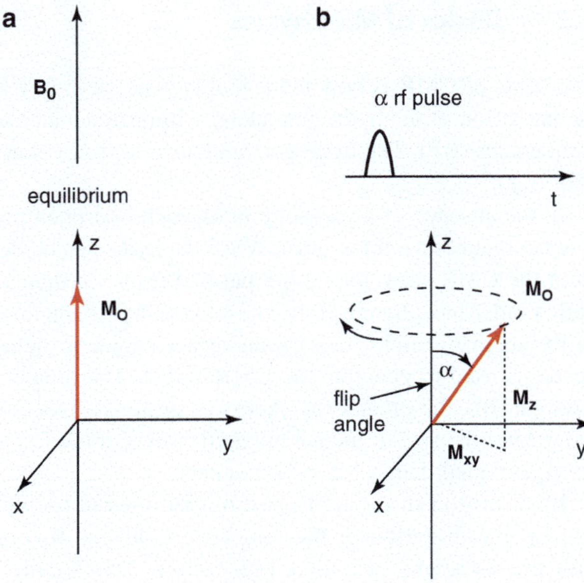

Fig. 1.3 When the radiofrequency is applied, the net magnetization begins to move away from its alignment along the axis of the main magnetic field (conventionally defined as z-axis). The greater the amount of applied energy, the greater will be the angle (flip angle) that the net magnetization makes with the B0 field (from J Cardiovasc Magn Reson. 2010 Nov 30;12:71 open access)

(or resonate) at this characteristic frequency. The constant in the Larmor equation is known as the gyromagnetic ratio and has a value that is characteristic for a particular nucleus (42.6 MHz/T for the proton). If a radiofrequency (emitted by radiofrequency transmitter coil) with the same frequency of the precession is applied, the hydrogen nuclei can be stimulated to flip perpendicularly to the direction of the main magnetic field (usually 1.5 or 3.0 tesla in clinical CMR machines).

When the radiofrequency is applied, the net magnetization begins to move away from its alignment along the axis of the main magnetic field (conventionally defined as z-axis). The greater the amount of applied energy, the greater will be the angle (flip angle) that the net magnetization makes with the B0 field (see Fig. 1.3).

Such radiofrequency (RF) pulses are named excitation pulses. After the application of the radiofrequency, the net magnetization has two components: (1) one component is parallel to the z-axis (Mz, also known as longitudinal component in Fig. 1.3) and (2) one component within the x-y axes (Mxy, also known as transverse component in Fig. 1.3). In CMR there are 90° RF pulses that are able to transfer all the magnetization on the transverse plane (xy plane) leaving no component on the longitudinal plane (z-axis). Such 90° RF pulses are named as saturation pulses. They provide the largest possible transverse magnetization and thus higher signal and better image quality but cannot be repeated as rapidly as a RF pulse with a smaller flip angle since the z-component of magnetization requires time to recover. RF pulses inducing a smaller flip angle (less than 90°) are presented by the symbol α, or with the specific angle (e.g. 30°), such pulses produce a smaller MR signal than a 90° RF pulse but can be repeated quicker than 90° RF pulses. A 180° RF pulse can be given when the net magnetization is already on the xy plane and then to flip the magnetization through 180 °C on the xy plane (refocusing pulse) or to invert the net longitudinal magnetization (inversion pulse; see Fig. 1.4).

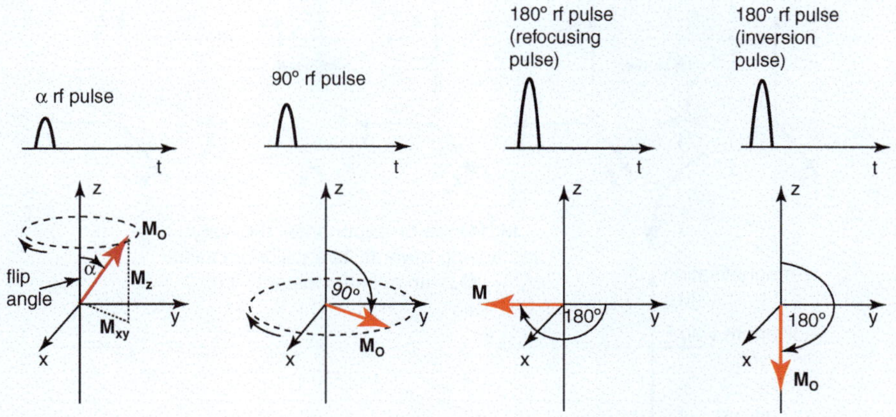

Fig. 1.4 Different RF pulses with different flip angles: (1) less than 90°, (2) excitatory 90° RF pulse, (3) 180° RF refocusing pulse on transverse plane and (4) 180° RF inversion pulse (from J Cardiovasc Magn Reson. 2010 Nov 30;12:71 open access)

The refocusing pulse is used in spin-echo sequences to reverse the loss of coherence in the transverse magnetization caused by magnetic field inhomogeneities. The inversion pulse does not generate a signal but is used as a magnetization preparation pulse (e.g. black-blood preparation sequence; see later in the chapter).

After excitation produced by the application of the RF pulse, protons tend to return to their basal state with alignment parallel to the main basal magnetic field. Such process of return back to the original state is named *relaxation*. There are two distinct types of relaxation:

1. *Longitudinal relaxation or T1 relaxation*: process of recovery of the original magnetization along the z-axis (also named saturation recovery after a 90° RF pulse)
2. *Transverse relaxation or T2 relaxation*: process of decay of the magnetization along the x-y axis

In human tissues the transverse or T2 relaxation occurs faster than the longitudinal or T1 magnetization. Both processes occur at the same time as exponential processes.

The longitudinal or T1 relaxation is described by an exponential curve where T1 is the time at which the magnetization has recovered to 63% of its value at equilibrium (Fig. 1.5).

Such return to the basal longitudinal magnetization occurs faster when hydrogen nuclei are able to release energy and go back to their basal state. Lipid molecules are especially faster and fat has shorter T1 relaxation time compared to muscle and water. Water and watery tissue (edematous tissue) has long T1 relaxation time since the energy exchange is not favoured.

The transverse or T2 relaxation is also described by an exponential curve, where T2 is the time at which the net transverse magnetization has decayed to 37% of its initial value after the 90° RF pulse (Fig. 1.6). The T2 relaxation is

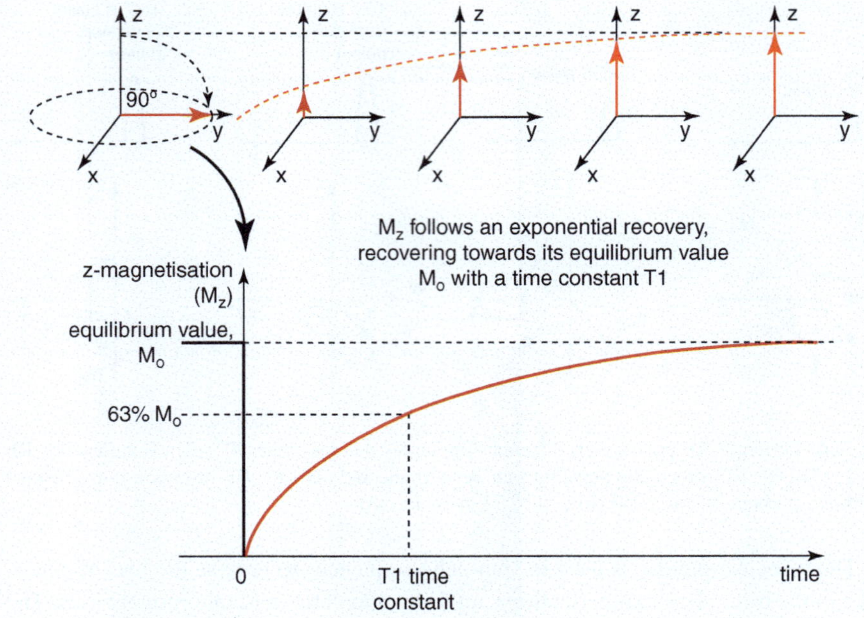

Fig. 1.5 Longitudinal or T1 relaxation according to an exponential curve (from J Cardiovasc Magn Reson. 2010 Nov 30;12:71 open access)

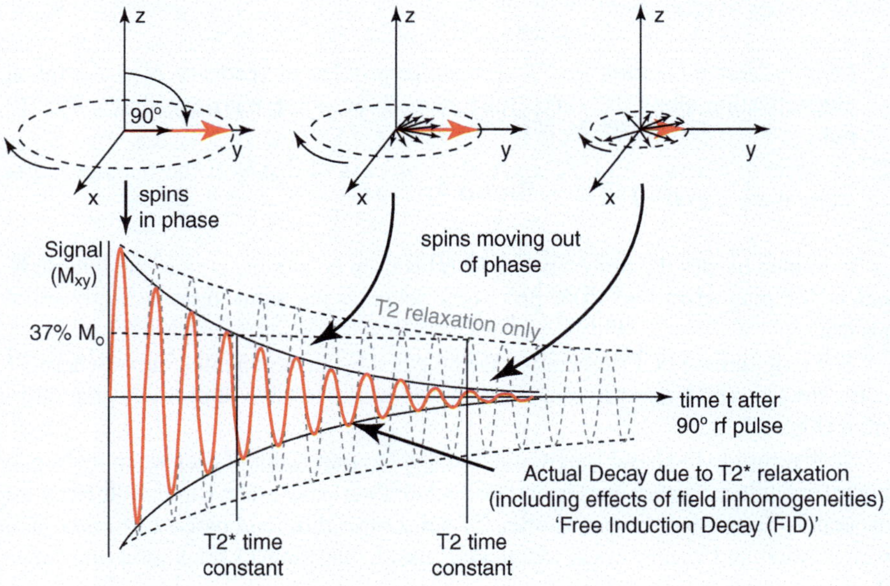

Fig. 1.6 Transverse relaxation or T2 relaxation according to an exponential curve (from J Cardiovasc Magn Reson. 2010 Nov 30;12:71 open access)

faster if there are more spin-to-spin interactions (usually this occurs more commonly for fat and muscle rather than water since free water contains small molecules that are relatively far apart and quickly moving). The amplitude of the transverse magnetization decays as protons move out of phase with one another. The resultant decaying signal is named the free induction decay (FID). This is the simple way to get a MR signal, but it is affected by gradient magnetic field applied to allow space encoding, and thus in clinical application the signal is acquired in a different way (see the following paragraph on how MR signal is generated).

Since inhomogeneities of the magnetic field due to tissue composition (e.g. presence of iron) can accelerate the signal decay by increased spin-to-spin interaction, the real T2 time, which occurs with the effects of such magnetic field inhomogeneities, is named T2*, and this relaxation is named T2* relaxation. The study of T2* is especially useful for the evaluation of iron overload. The possible effect of magnetic field inhomogeneities can be reversed by a 180° refocusing pulse (Fig. 1.6).

1.3 How the MR Signal Is Generated and Basic CMR Sequences

The MR signal is generated from the relaxation phenomenon. Since magnetic field gradients used to localize the MR signal may affect the simple free induction decay (FID), the MR signal is generated in the form of an echo. The two more common types of echo are gradient and spin echoes. The RM signal is called "echo" since it is a transient RM signal that reappears after the disappearance of the initial signal induced by the first excitatory RF pulse.

1.3.1 Gradient Echoes

Gradient echoes are generated by the application of a 90° RF pulse that gives origin to a T2* relaxation followed by the application of two subsequent magnetic field gradients in opposite direction: the first magnetic gradient causes a rapid de-phasing of the transverse magnetization (the FID signal rapidly drop to zero), while the second magnetic gradient echo applied in the opposite direction causes the rephasing of the signal with the generation of a MR echo signal named gradient echo at the echo time (TE; Fig. 1.7). The second gradient echo is maintained for a time equivalent to twice the time of the first gradient echo and thus causing the FID signal to de-phase to zero. The amplitude of the gradient echo depends on T2* relaxation and the chosen TE. The time from the RF pulse to the maximum amplitude of the echo is known as the echo time, TE.

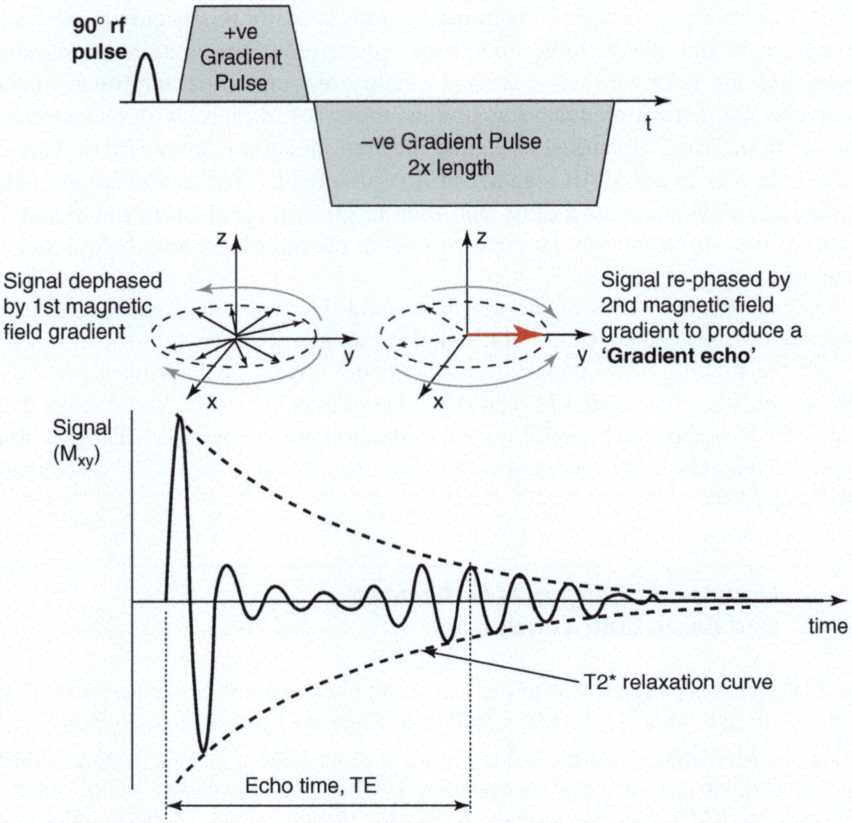

Fig. 1.7 Gradient-echo sequence (see text for explanation; from J Cardiovasc Magn Reson. 2010 Nov 30;12:71 open access)

1.3.2 Spin Echoes

Spin echoes are generated by a 90° RF excitatory pulse followed by a 180° RF refocusing pulse applied at the specific time equal to TE/2 (Fig. 1.8). The FID following the T2 relaxation time (since the magnetic inhomogeneities are compensated by the refocusing RF pulse) has the maximal amplitude at the echo time (TE). After reaching its maximal intensity at the TE time, the signal de-phases following T2* relaxation. The signal produced by this MR sequence is called spin echo. The spin-echo signal is greater than the gradient-echo signal and less affected by magnetic field inhomogeneities. On the contrary, if the aim of the MR sequence is to detect iron overload, gradient-echo signals are needed for this evaluation.

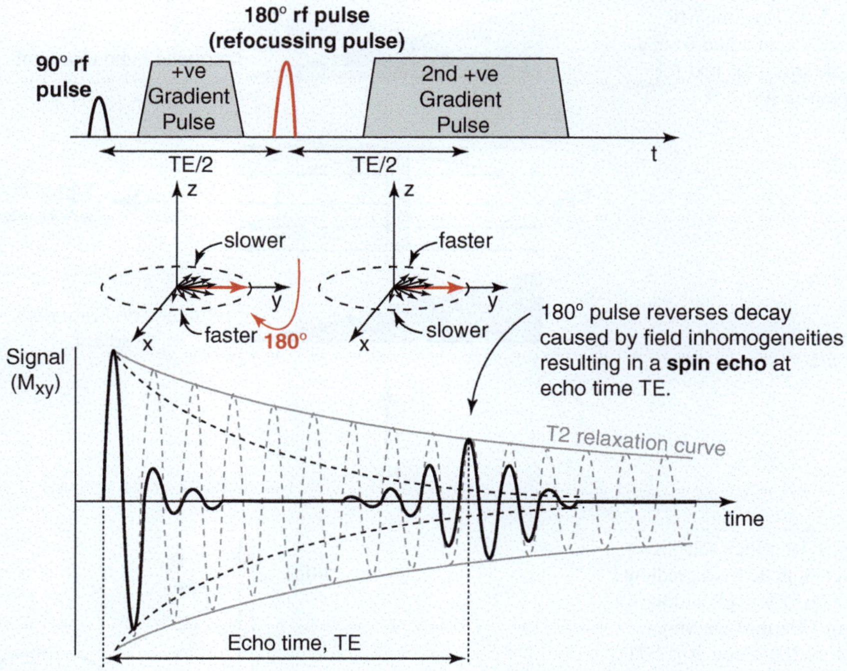

Fig. 1.8 Spin-echo sequence (see text for explanation; from J Cardiovasc Magn Reson. 2010 Nov 30;12:71 open access)

1.4 Spatial Encoding and Image Reconstruction

Spatial encoding in CMR is complicated and to provide a simplified vision of it, we will simplify and summarize the main concepts.

Basically, in order to generate a signal for a specific slice of the body, a magnetic field gradient is applied (Fig. 1.9). Such magnetic gradient creates also a gradient of precession frequency: in Fig. 1.10 the precession frequency will be higher towards the head compared to the feet in the scanner. With an applied RF with a selected frequency, only a selected tissue slide will be excited by the RF and will generate a signal from a single slice, thus creating the basing for a 2D CMR signal.

This magnetic gradient is created by a gradient coil in the scanner (see additional description later in Chap. 2).

Spatial encoding is reached by (1) slice selection (Fig. 1.10), (2) phase encoding (Fig. 1.11) and (3) frequency encoding (Fig. 1.11).

Since there are three sets of gradient coils, perpendicular to each other, it is possible to create gradients in three dimensions (spatial encoding gradients) and having

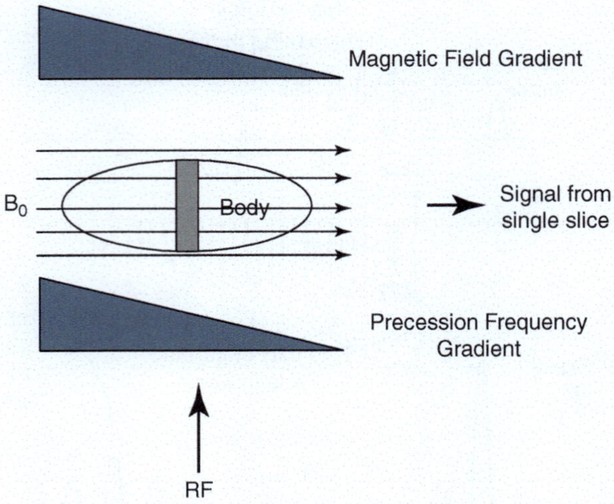

Fig. 1.9 How the MR signal is generated from a single slice (see text for explanation)

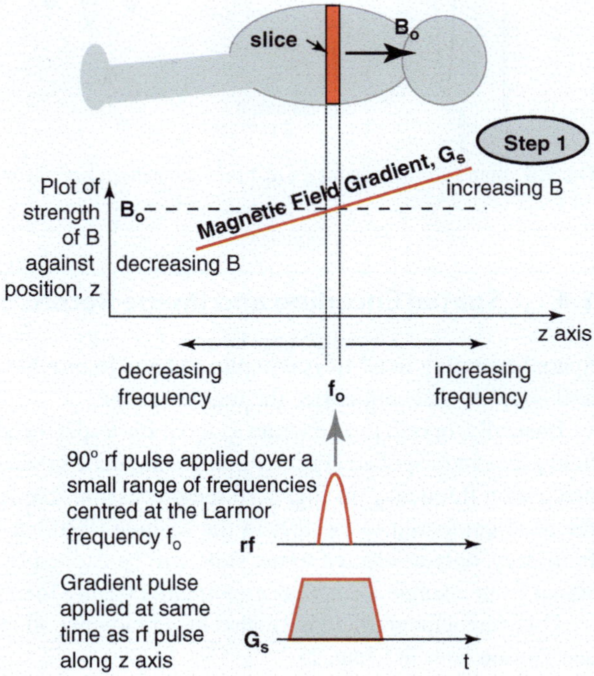

Fig. 1.10 Slice selection and magnetic field gradient (see text for explanation; from J Cardiovasc Magn Reson. 2010 Nov 30;12:71 open access)

2D imaging in any spatial plane in the scanner (unrestrictive imaging planes that can be generated in CMR).

In summary, to localize the MR signal in three dimensions, three separate magnetic field gradients are applied in a three-step process.

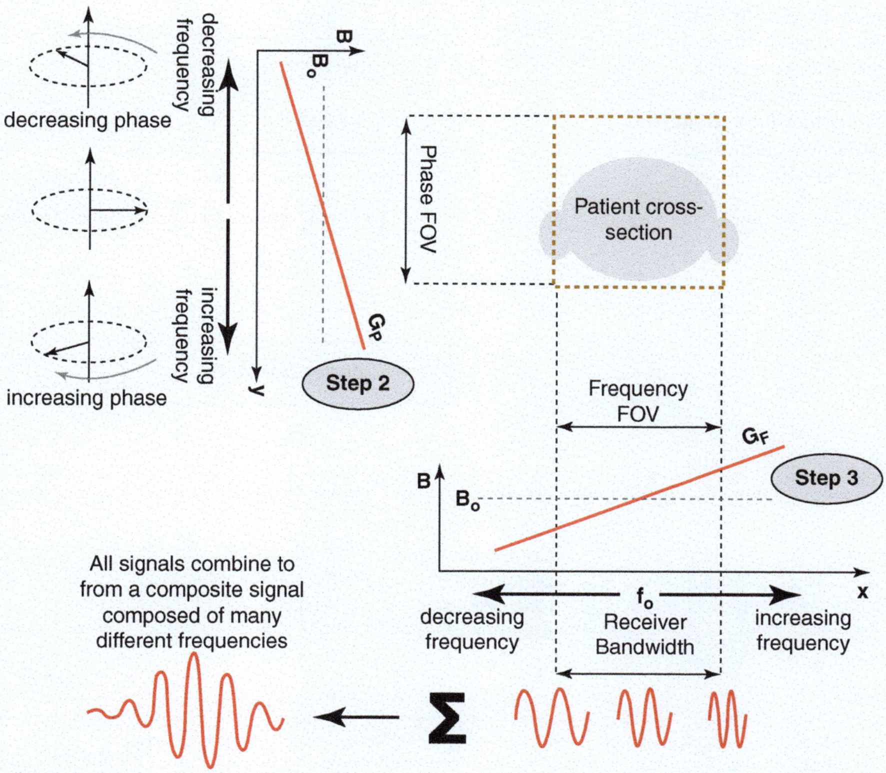

Fig. 1.11 Spatial encoding by: (Step 2) phase encoding and (Step 3) frequency encoding (from J Cardiovasc Magn Reson. 2010 Nov 30;12:71 open access)

The MR image is reconstructed using an algorithm, known as a two-dimensional (2D) Fourier transform. This is applied to the resultant signals to decode the contributions from different locations based on their frequency and the change in phase with each phase encoding step (Fig. 1.12). In order to acquire sufficient information for image reconstruction, the pulse sequence is repeated a number of times with an increment in the strength or slope of the phase encoding (Fig. 1.13). The time interval between each repetition is known as repetition time (TR). A number of repetitions (Np) are needed for each image, and the image acquisition time is related to both the number of repetitions (Np) and the repetition time (TR).

$$\text{Image acquisition time} = \text{Np} \times \text{TR}$$

A better spatial resolution requires more Np and thus a longer acquisition time.

All the rough data acquired by the CMR scan are collected in the *k-space*. The *k-space* can be simply defined as a box where the rough data are collected and

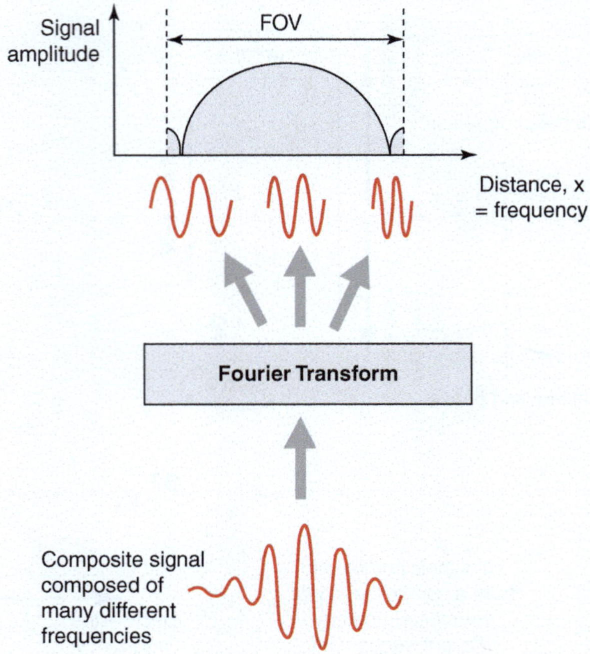

Fig. 1.12 The MR image is reconstructed using an algorithm, known as a two-dimensional (2D) Fourier transform (from J Cardiovasc Magn Reson. 2010 Nov 30;12:71 open access)

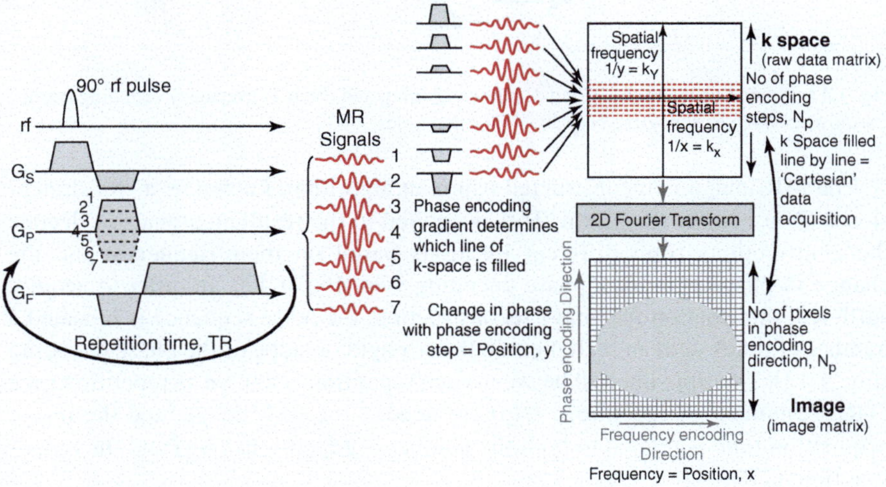

Fig. 1.13 In order to acquire sufficient information for image reconstruction, the pulse sequence is repeated a number of times with an increment in the strength or slope of the phase encoding (from J Cardiovasc Magn Reson. 2010 Nov 30;12:71 open access)

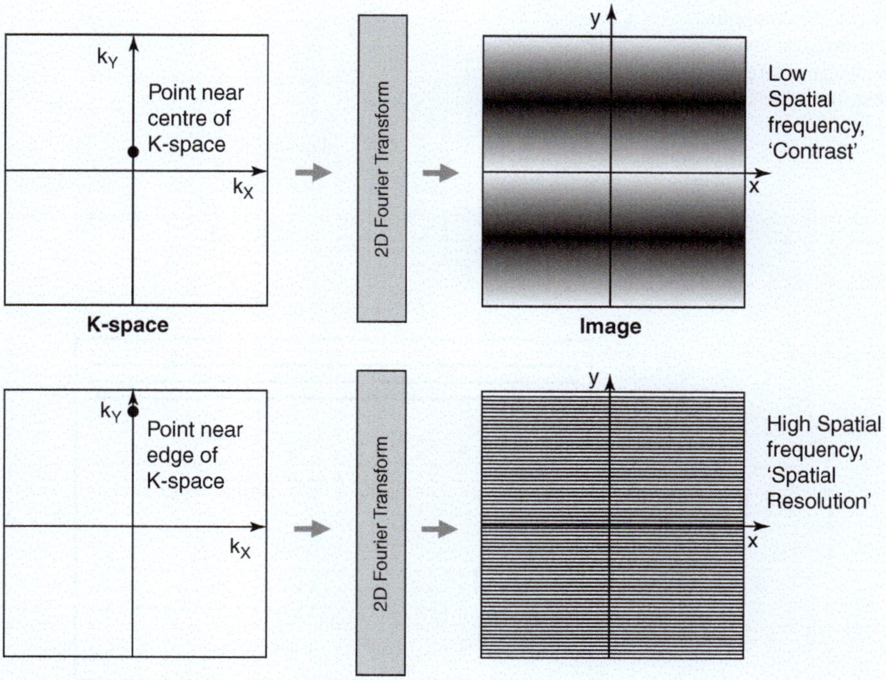

Fig. 1.14 The row data in the k-space are frequencies. The low-frequency data (peak to peak far away) are contained near the centre of the k-space, and they contribute to the definition of the image contrast and gross attributes, while high frequencies (peak to peak closer) are at the edges of the k-space and contribute to the fine details and the edges, defining the spatial resolution of the image (from J Cardiovasc Magn Reson. 2010 Nov 30;12:71 open access)

processed and the image is created by this processing (Figs. 1.14 and 1.15). The row data in the k-space are frequencies. The low-frequency data (peak to peak far away) are contained near the centre of the k-space, and they contribute to the definition of the image contrast and gross attributes, while high frequencies (peak to peak closer) are at the edges of the k-space and contribute to the fine details and the edges, defining the spatial resolution of the image. In order to acquire the MR image, all frequencies must be represented.

There are different methods to fill the k-space. The simplest is line by line (Cartesian acquisition) and it is adopted by the majority of cardiovascular applications. Nevertheless there are also other ways of filling the k-space (e.g. radial, spiral) with advantages and disadvantages. For instance, it may be required to quickly get contrast information after injection of the contrast media (angiography application): in this case the filling of the k-space starts from the centre and moves outwards (low frequencies near the centre of the k-space contribute especially to the image contrast).

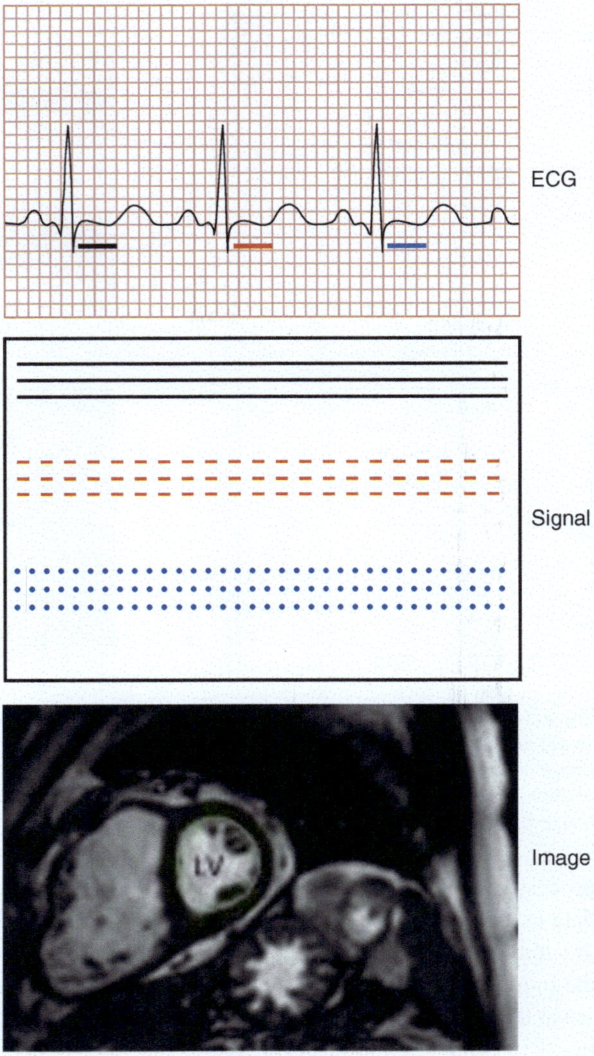

Fig. 1.15 Simplified summary on how MR image is generated (see text for explanation)

1.5 Tissue Characterization by Cardiac Magnetic Resonance (CMR)

CMR is able to generate images with different contrasts from different soft tissue (e.g. fat, muscle) in the same image. Such contrast is generated by the way different tissues recover from the original excitation by RF.

Fat has a short T1 compared with water; thus on T1-weighted images with appropriate image acquisition, the signal intensity from fat is higher than from muscle tissue and water, and fat appears brighter (Fig. 1.16). Gadolinium contrast agents

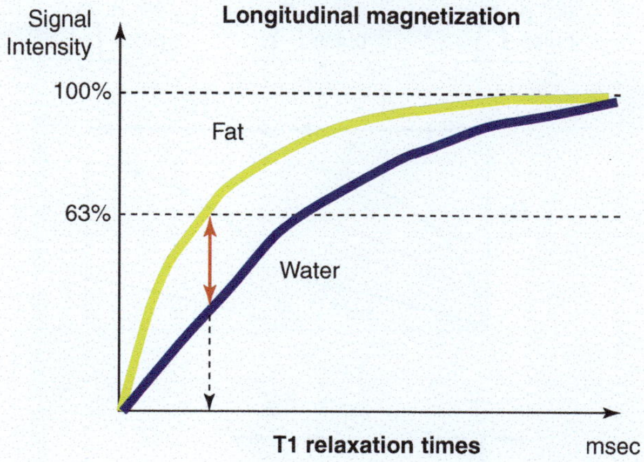

Fig. 1.16 Fat has a short T1 compared with water; thus on T1-weighted images with appropriate image acquisition, the signal intensity from fat is higher than from muscle tissue and water, and fat appears brighter

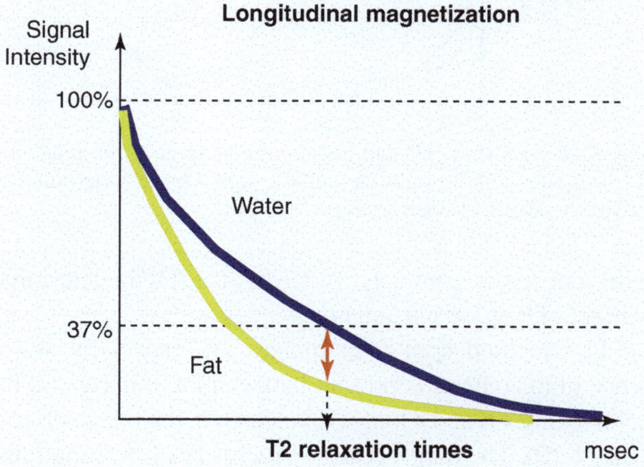

Fig. 1.17 In T2-weighted images, the acquisition with a sufficiently long time allows good discrimination between watery tissue (e.g. edematous myocardium) and normal myocardium having shorter T2; thus edema is brighter in these sequences

have the property to shorten T1 relaxation times; thus if gadolinium is present in the extracellular space (e.g. myocardial fibrosis), the fibrotic myocardium has a shorten T1 and appears brighter on T1-weighted images compared to normal myocardium.

In T2-weighted images, the acquisition with a sufficiently long time allows good discrimination between watery tissue (e.g. edematous myocardium) and normal myocardium having shorter T2; thus edema is brighter in these sequences (Fig. 1.17).

In spin-echo sequences, the image contrast may be T1-weighted or T2-weighted according to the selection of TE and TR times.

If a short TR and a short TE is selected, the image on a spin-echo sequence will be T1-weighted with a bright fat and low signal from static fluid (see Figs. 1.16 and 1.18). A short TR means that the subsequent 90° excitatory RF will occur when tissues with short T1 (e.g. fat) have recovered more than tissues with a long T1 (e.g. muscle and even more for fluids); thus the subsequent transverse magnetization will be greater for tissues with a short T1 (e.g. fat) that will appear with a higher signal intensity (that is brighter). The short TE limits the effect of T2 relaxation on the

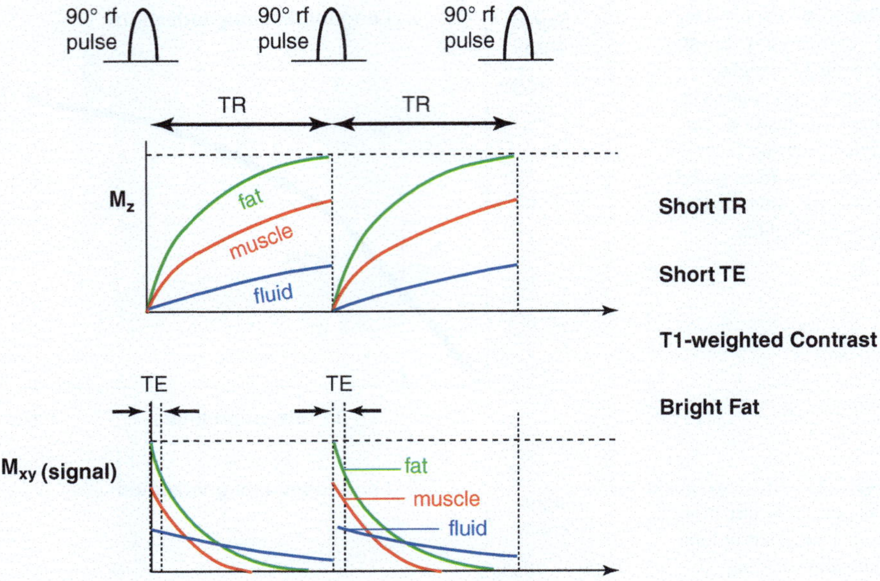

Fig. 1.18 If a short TR and a short TE is selected, the image on a spin-echo sequence will be T1-weighted with a bright fat and low signal from static fluid (from J Cardiovasc Magn Reson. 2010 Nov 30;12:71 open access)

different tissue contrasts. In CMR, the TR is determined by the heart rate of the patient (TR = 1 × RR interval).

T1-weighted spin-echo images are especially suitable for anatomic imaging since high contrast is present between fat, muscle and fluid.

If a long TR and a long TE is selected, the image on spin echo will be T2-weighted (Fig. 1.19). The long TR allows recovery of the longitudinal magnetization and thus limits the contrast due to a different T1 relaxation, while a long TE allows more decay of the transverse magnetization. Thus tissues with a long T2 (e.g. fluids) will be discriminated from tissues with a shorter T2 (e.g. muscle and fat). These images are characterized by bright fluids and are especially useful to depict fluid collections and edema. In these sequences the TR time is set to 2 or 3 times the RR interval.

In spin-echo imaging, there is a black-blood contrast due to the moving blood since blood that received the 90° RF pulse washes out of the slice during the TE/2 before the 180°RF pulse (see Fig. 1.20).

If a long TR (T1 relaxation differences are not visible) and a short TE (to minimize the tissue contrast due to T2 relaxation) are selected, the image on spin echo will be proton density-weighted (Fig. 1.21). The result is high signal from all tissues that can be used for anatomical imaging when soft tissue discrimination is not needed.

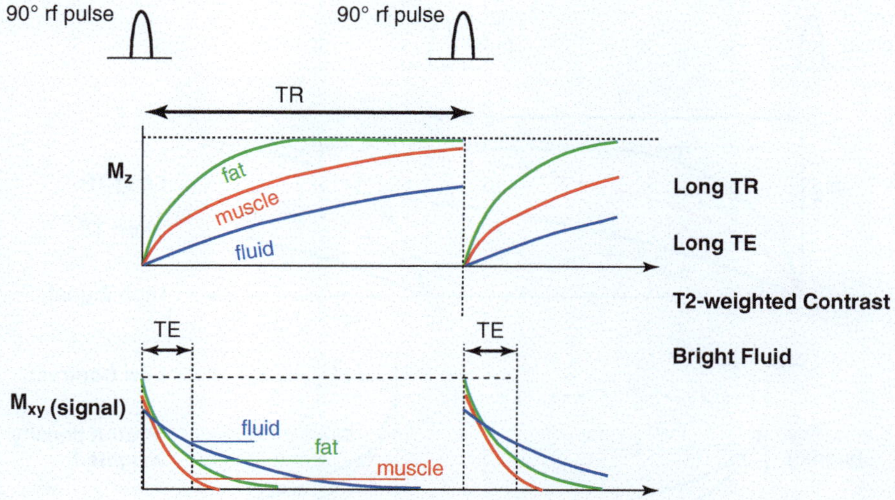

Fig. 1.19 If a long TR and a long TE is selected, the image on spin echo will be T2-weighted (Fig. 1.19). The long TR allows recovery of the longitudinal magnetization and thus limits the contrast due to a different T1 relaxation, while a long TE allows more decay of the transverse magnetization. Thus tissues with a long T2 (e.g. fluids) will be discriminated from tissues with a shorter T2 (e.g. muscle and fat) (from J Cardiovasc Magn Reson. 2010 Nov 30;12:71 open access)

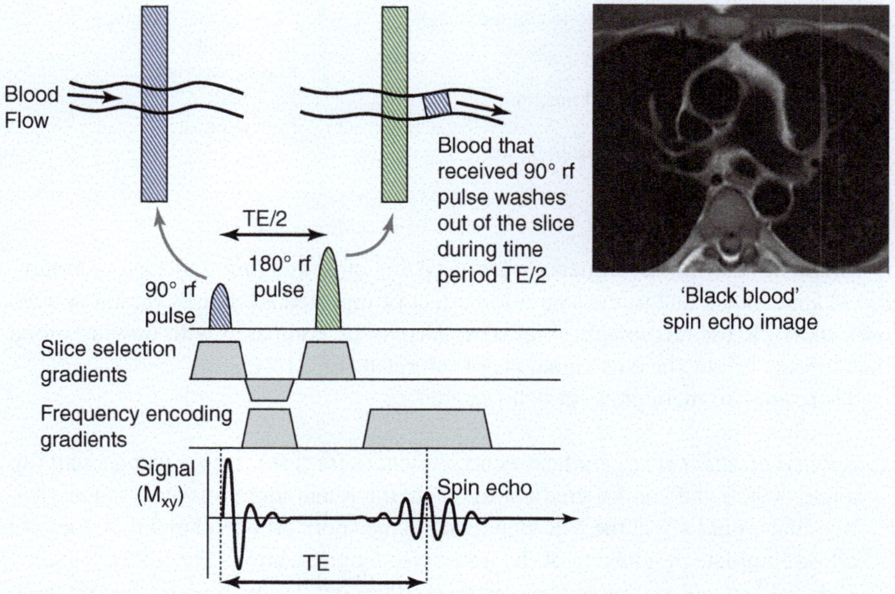

Fig. 1.20 In spin-echo imaging, there is a black-blood contrast due to the moving blood since blood that received the 90° RF pulse washes out of the slice during the TE/2 before the 180°RF pulse (from J Cardiovasc Magn Reson. 2010 Nov 30;12:71 open access)

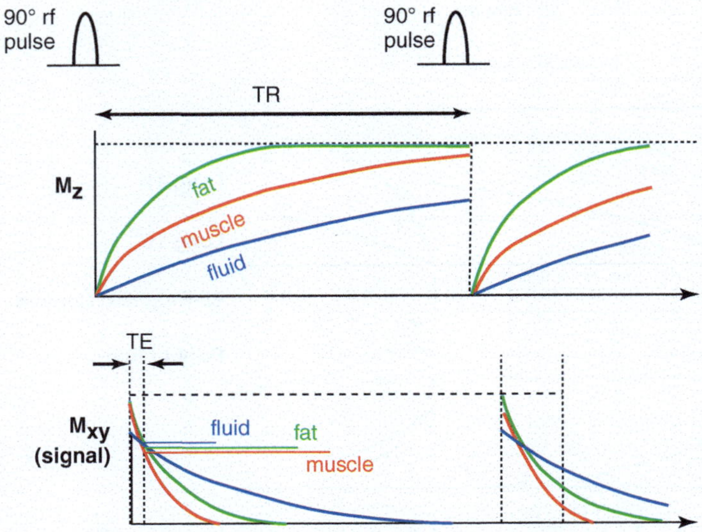

Fig. 1.21 If a long TR (T1 relaxation differences are not visible) and a short TE (to minimize the tissue contrast due to T2 relaxation) are selected, the image on spin echo will be proton density-weighted (from J Cardiovasc Magn Reson. 2010 Nov 30;12:71 open access)

	Short TE	Long TE
Long TR	Proton density-weighted imaging Good SNR No contrast	T2-weighted imaging Low signal from fat Fluids are bright
Short TR	T1-weighted imaging Bright fat Low signal from fluids	Poor SNR Poor contrast

SNR signal-to-noise ratio

Gradient-echo pulse sequences are used for cine imaging and have a bright-blood appearance due to the saturation effect of repeated RF pulses (gradient echo uses short TR for fast imaging) on stationary tissue compared with flowing blood that appears bright since its signal is not saturated (Fig. 1.21).

There are two main gradient-echo sequences:

1. *Spoiled gradient echo*: gradient-echo sequences for fast imaging using small flip angle (<90°) and spoiler gradient to delete the remaining transverse magnetization that would affect the MR signal due to the short TR (<400 ms) that does not allow complete de-phasing of the transverse magnetization (Fig. 1.22).
2. *Balanced steady-state free precession*: gradient-echo sequences for fast imaging using small flip angle (<90 °C) but no spoiler gradients so that the remnant magnetization is maintained and signal can sum up after a number of repetition

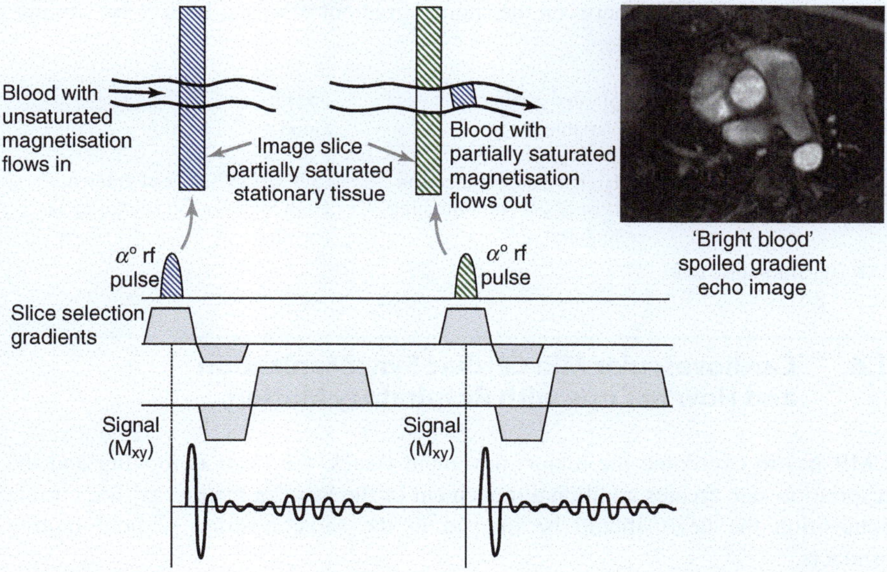

Fig. 1.22 Bright-blood spoiled gradient-echo sequences for cine imaging (from J Cardiovasc Magn Reson. 2010 Nov 30;12:71 open access)

reaching a steady state that give a much larger signal than spoiled gradient echo. The MR signal is acquired at TE = TR/2 so that the acquired image is related to the T2/T1 ratio.

A comparison of the main differences between spin-echo and gradient-echo sequences is reported in the following table:

	Spin echo	Gradient echo (spoiled)	Gradient echo (bSSFP)
Flip angle	90°	<90° (5–40°)	<90° (50–70°)
180° refocusing pulse	Yes	No	NO
Contrast weighting	T1, T2, proton density	T1, T2*	T2/T1 ratio
Short TR	No (400–800 ms)	Yes (3–400 ms)	Yes (3–5 ms)
Signal from blood flow	Dark	Bright	Bright
Cardiac application	Anatomical imaging and tissue characterization	Fast cine imaging, flow imaging, contrast-enhanced MR angiography, T2*-weighted imaging (iron overload)	Fast cine imaging

The main differences between the spoiled gradient echo and bSSFP are summarized in the following table:

Image feature	Spoiled gradient echo	bSSFP
Blood to myocardium contrast	Variable	Good – T2/T1 ratio
Flow sensitivity	High – can visualize jets	Low – uses balanced gradients
Image quality	Low SNR – no shimming required	High SNR – good shimming is required

SNR signal-to-noise ratio

1.6 Cardiovascular MR: Cardiac Synchronization and How to Cope with Respiratory Motion

CMR has to overcome the major movement issues: the heart is moving and the respiration also creates additional movement of the heart in the thorax. For correct acquisition the heart should be imaged in the same position without motion artefacts.

In order to overcome the problem of cardiac motion, the image acquisition should be fast with a TR as short as possible. In order to preserve an acceptable degree of image quality, cardiac synchronization is needed. Cardiac synchronization is achieved by using the ECG signal obtained by ECG pads. The R wave is recognized, and MR data acquisition is synchronized so that MR signals are acquired over multiple beats synchronizing the signal acquisition at a particular time of the cardiac cycle.

The image acquisition is performed when the heart is not moving acquiring different pieces of information in different heartbeats as depicted in the example in Fig. 1.23 (concept of segmented k-space).

Two types of cardiac images can be acquired: still images obtained at a single point and cine imaging by acquisition at multiple points through the cardiac cycle.

Respiratory motion may affect the quality of the acquired images. This issue can be managed by three methods: (1) respiratory compensation methods (respiratory gating), (2) cardiac synchronized fast imaging and breath-hold and (3) ultrafast (single-shot) imaging techniques. Respiratory activity is monitored by a respiratory bellows pad.

The issue of respiration motion can be managed with three different approaches:

1. Fast imaging with breath-holding (most common)
2. Respiratory gating
3. Real-time (ultrafast) image acquisition without breath-holding

In CMR the issue of respiratory motion is usually managed through breath-holding. The patient is invited to stop breathing for up to 15 s in order to allow CMR image acquisition. Since sick patients have difficulties to stop breathing for >15 s, one challenge of CMR is to speed the acquisition time.

Fig. 1.23 MR imaging: from signal to image (see text for explanation)

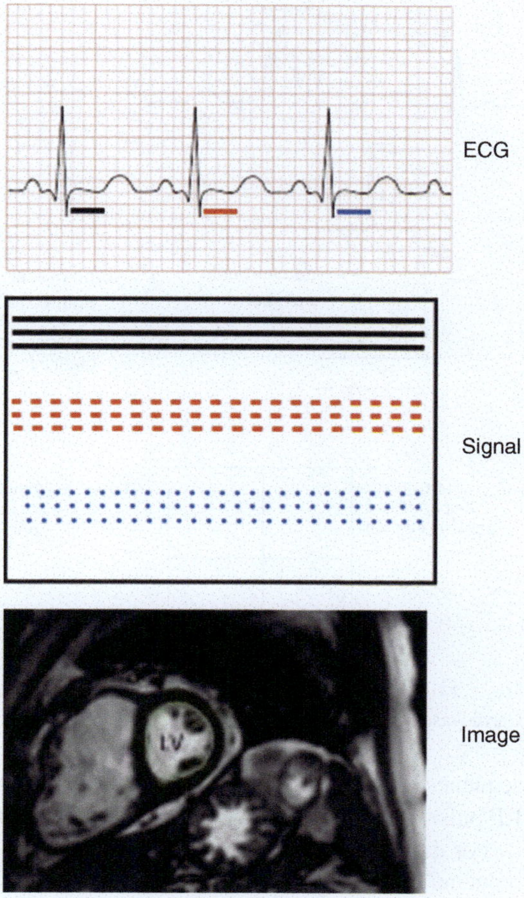

Respiratory gating is performed by monitoring the respiratory activity of the patients, and data can be acquired only if coming from a prespecified time (usually end expiration since it is usually the longer part of the respiratory cycle for each patient). More complex and accurate method includes the use of navigator echoes such as in coronary MR angiography (see later in the chapter).

1.7 Common Cardiac MR Imaging Techniques

1.7.1 Still Imaging (Black-Blood Anatomical Imaging)

Such imaging technique is based on triggering: ECG synchronization is obtained by the detection of the R wave with MR signal acquisition at the prespecified time after the R wave (trigger). Commonly adopted sequences are turbo or fast spin echo (for Philips and Siemens, the sequence is named TSE = turbo spin echo; for GE the

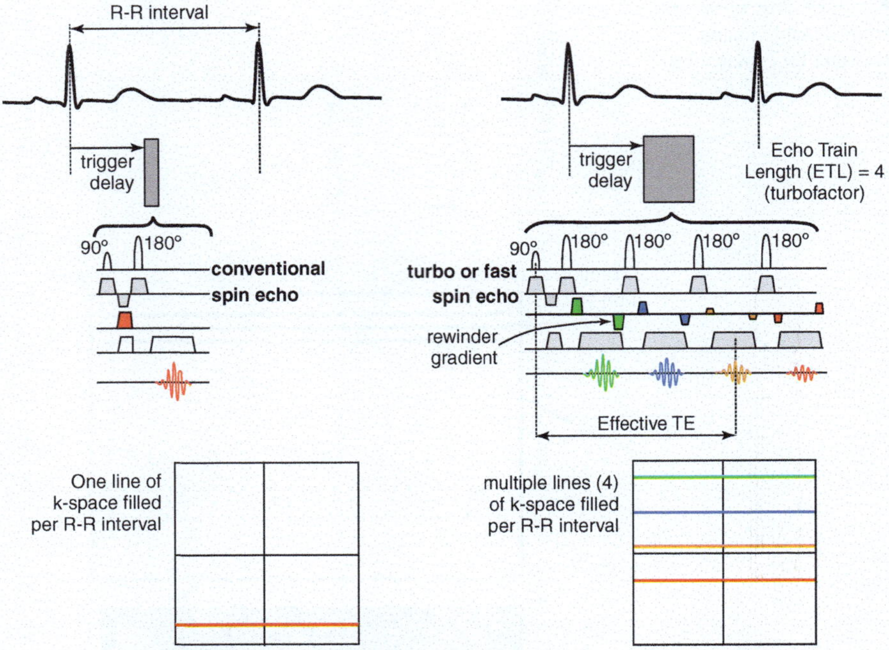

Fig. 1.24 Conventional vs. turbo or fast spin-echo sequences (see text for explanation; from J Cardiovasc Magn Reson. 2010 Nov 30;12:71 open access)

sequence is named FSE = fast spin echo). The sequence is based on multiple 180° RF pulses after the initial 90° RF pulse (Fig. 1.24).

For each excitatory RF pulse, multiple lines of the k-space are acquired, thus reducing acquisition time. The number of echoes acquired for each excitatory RF pulse is named echo train length (ETL) or turbofactor. Usually an ETL of 15–20 is necessary to acquire the image within a breath-hold. In black-blood anatomical imaging, dark-blood contrast is increased by the use of a double-inversion preparatory pulse. This preparation consists of RF inversion pulses followed by a delay prior to the 90°excitatory RF: the first pulse is not slice selective, while the second is slice selective so that if an appropriate time delay (TI = inversion recovery time) is waited before the 90° excitatory RF pulse, the signal from the blood in the selected tissue slice is black (Fig. 1.25). This TI time is calculated to provide the best blood suppression depending on the heart rate (usually TI is 400–600 ms). Essentially this sequence allows selective acquisition of a MR signal for a selected slice of tissue since blood is flowing out of the slice and the signal from moving blood is low, thus providing contrast and the basis for black-blood anatomical imaging.

1.7.2 Cine Imaging

Cine imaging is adopted for evaluation of cardiac function by wall motion analysis and volumes estimation and is based on bright-blood cine imaging by gradient-echo

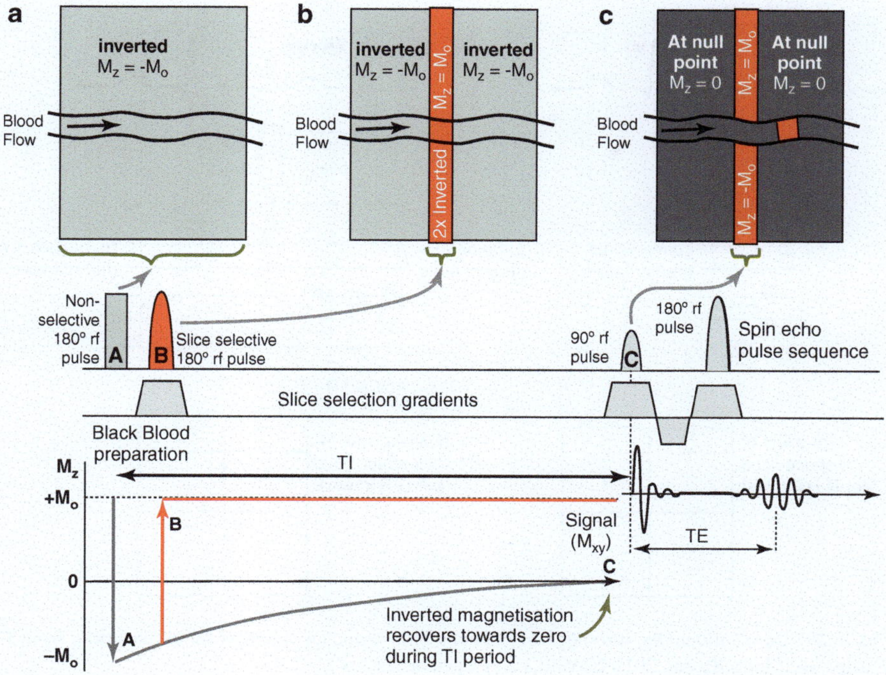

Fig. 1.25 Black-blood preparation (see text for explanation; from J Cardiovasc Magn Reson. 2010 Nov 30;12:71 open access)

techniques that acquire the images at different phases of the cardiac cycle and are put together in a movie.

Cine imaging requires fast TR and uses gradient-echo pulse sequences by acceleration of the sequence through repetitions of the low flip angle RF pulse to generate multiple gradient echoes and acquisition of multiple lines of the k-space within each cardiac cycle instead of one line as in conventional gradient-echo imaging (Fig. 1.26).

The number of lines that are acquired for each shot is named in a different way according to the manufacturer: views per segment (GE), turbofactor (Philips) and no of segments (Siemens). Increasing the number of k-space that are acquired reduces the scan time but increases the acquisition window of each cardiac cycle, thus reducing the number of cardiac cycle that can be imaged and temporal resolution.

Accelerated gradient-echo imaging can be applied to both spoiled gradient-echo and bSSFP sequences and has different names according to the manufacturer (see table).

	GE	Philips	Siemens
Fast spoiled gradient echo	Fast spoiled GRASS (FSPGR)	T1-weighted turbo field echo (T1-TFE)	TurboFLASH (TFL)
Balanced steady-state free precession (bSSFP)	Fast imaging employing steady-state acquisition (FIESTA)	Balanced turbo field echo (TFE)	Segmented true FISP

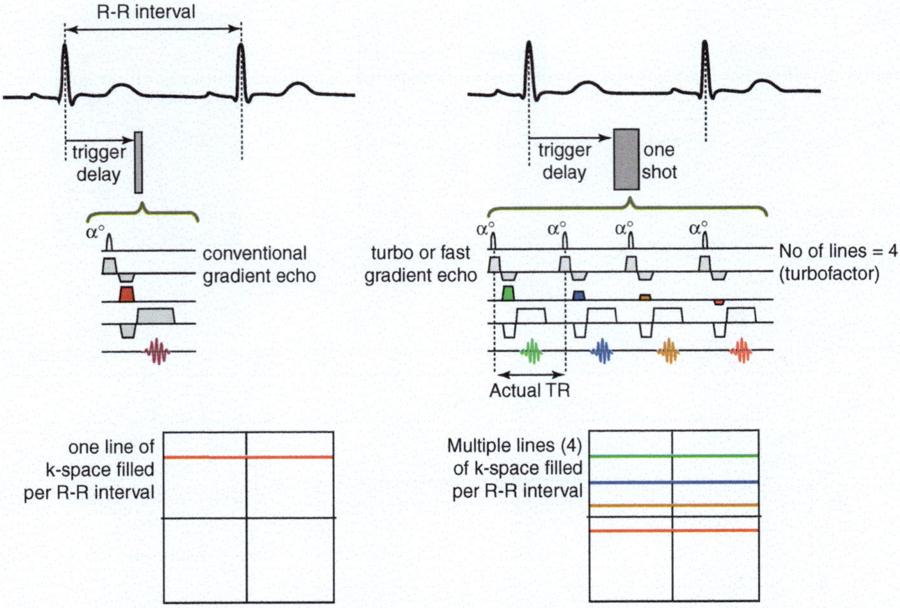

Fig. 1.26 Conventional vs. turbo or fast gradient-echo sequence (see text for explanation; from J Cardiovasc Magn Reson. 2010 Nov 30;12:71 open access)

Cine imaging requires cardiac synchronization and the acquisition of data from a single slice location at multiple points of the cardiac cycle with subsequent reconstruction. Each cardiac phase lasts a TR and TR time is short (Fig. 1.27).

It can be performed by:

1. *ECG triggering* initiating the data acquisition of the first cardiac phase immediately after the R wave and then stop before the next R wave that is detected, so that a part of the cardiac cycle is missed.
2. *Retrospective ECG gating* with continuous recording and retrospective sorting of cardiac phase without any loss of last part of the cardiac cycle close to the R wave. It can be performed with small variations of the RR interval.

In patients with arrhythmias and consistent RR interval variations, although a possible correction of the variable RR time is possible by the option named *arrhythmia rejection*, there are two possibilities: (1) use of ECG triggering or (2) real-time acquisition at the expenses of temporal and spatial resolution.

At 1.5 tesla the balanced SSFP gradient-echo sequence is used for most functional imaging applications and volumetric assessments due to the high intrinsic contrast between blood and myocardium throughout the cardiac cycle. The spoiled

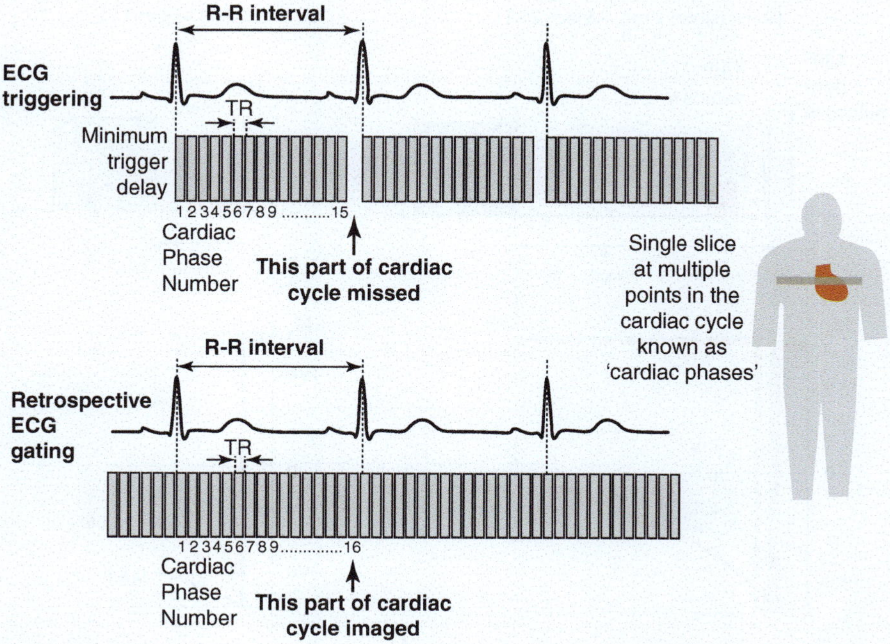

Fig. 1.27 ECG triggering and retrospective ECG gating (from J Cardiovasc Magn Reson. 2010 Nov 30;12:71 open access)

gradient-echo pulse sequence is often used for the assessment of flow jets and thus valvular heart diseases, due to its greater flow sensitivity (see table).

Cine imaging	Sequence	Clinical use
SSFP	FIESTA (GE) Balanced TFE (Philips) Segmented true FISP	Function (1.5 T), volumes measures
Spoiled gradient echo	FSPGR (GE) T1-TFE (Philips) TFL (Siemens)	Function (3 T), flow assessment and flow jets

1.7.3 T1- or T2-Weighted Black-Blood FSE/TSE Pulse Sequences

The classical technique for anatomical imaging of cardiac structure is based on black-blood preparation with the application of a 180° RF non-slice selective pulse that inverts the longitudinal magnetization of all tissues followed by a slice-selective 180° RF pulse that reverts the longitudinal magnetization in the tissues belonging to the slice of interest and then after a determined time (the inversion

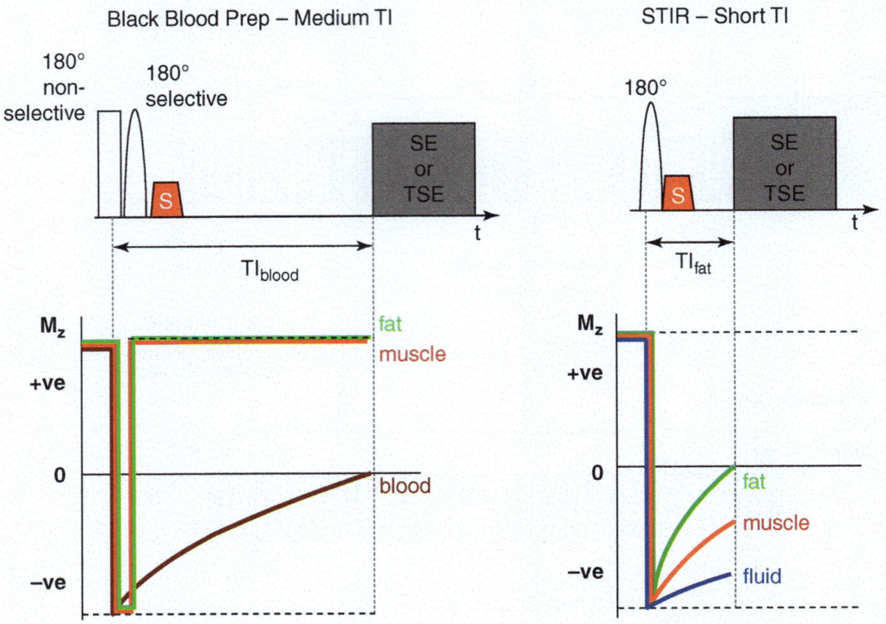

Fig. 1.28 Black-blood preparation and T1-weighted imaging vs. STIR T2-weighted imaging (see text for explanation; from J Cardiovasc Magn Reson. 2012 Sep 20;14:66)

time of the blood) the spin-echo pulse to generate the MR signal from the slice of interest (Fig. 1.28).

The Short TI Inversion Recovery (STIR) is a sequence where, after a slice-selective 180° RF pulse that inverts the longitudinal magnetization of the tissues, a short inversion time (TI) is chosen to null the signal from fat tissue (Fig. 1.28). For edema depiction a combined sequence with black-blood preparation is followed by a STIR sequence in order to suppress the signal from blood and fat. In this case a long TE is also chosen to have a T2-weighted imaging to allow the identification of edema as a bright signal (Fig. 1.29). This technique is also referred as T2-weighted STIR and is based on a triple inversion RF pulse.

1.7.4 Fat Suppression by Chemical Shift

Another way to get fat suppression is to use the slight difference of Larmor frequency of hydrogen nuclei in fat tissue compared to water molecules, also named as *chemical shift*. At 1.5 tesla, this difference is 220 Hz; thus if a 90° RF saturation pulse is applied at the Larmor frequency of fat as preparatory pulse, the signal from fat is suppressed in subsequent imaging. An efficacious suppression requires an adequate uniformity of the magnetic field. This frequency-selective method of fat suppression is also known as chemical shift selective (CHESS) imaging.

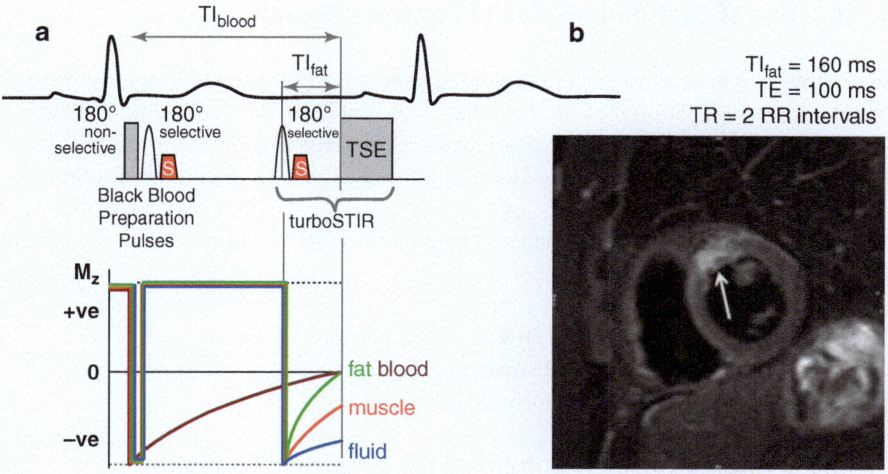

Fig. 1.29 T2-weighted STIR sequence and imaging (see text for additional explanation; from J Cardiovasc Magn Reson. 2012 Sep 20;14:66)

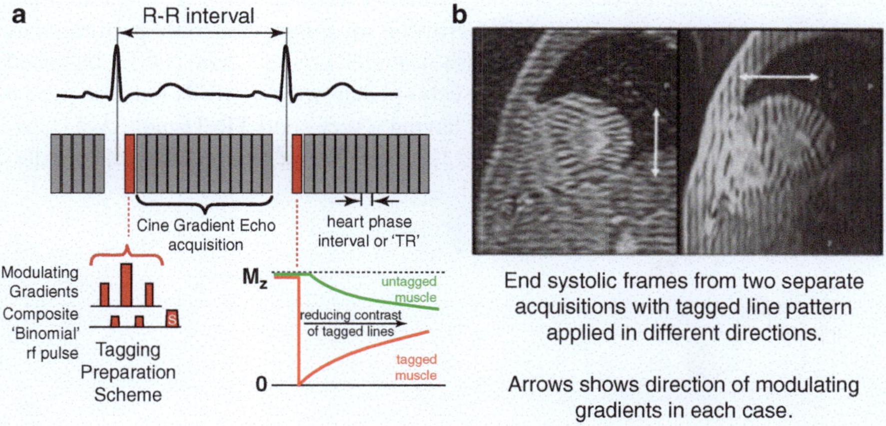

Fig. 1.30 Myocardial tagging sequence (see text for additional explanation; from J Cardiovasc Magn Reson. 2012 Sep 20;14:66)

1.7.5 Myocardial Tagging

The application of a net of non-selective preparatory RF pulses applied after the R wave (end diastole) allows myocardial tagging. This is commonly referred to as tagging or spatial modulation of magnetization (SPAMM). The magnetization pattern appears as a series of low-signal-intensity parallel lines across the image where the magnetization has been saturated. As the heart contracts through systole, the magnetization pattern deforms as it follows the contraction of the myocardial muscle (Fig. 1.30). This technique allows the detection of abnormality of myocardial contraction.

1.7.6 Use of Gadolinium-Based Contrast Agents

In cardiac magnetic resonance, contrast agents are based on gadolinium, a heavy metal with strong paramagnetic properties, that is able to reduce T1 time of tissues. Gadolinium-based contrast agents are extracellular since gadolinium cannot enter the cell membrane of intact cells. Gadolinium is a high toxic metal that is administrated as chelates.

In cardiac magnetic resonance, applications of contrast agents include especially:

1. Dynamic contrast-enhanced (DCE) cardiac perfusion imaging
2. Early and late gadolinium enhancement (LGE)
3. Magnetic resonance angiography (MRA)

1.7.6.1 Dynamic Contrast-Enhanced (DCE) Cardiac Perfusion Imaging

Contrast agent is injected intravenously and can be seen as signal enhancement in the right ventricular cavity (RV) followed by the left ventricular cavity (LV) and more gradually in the myocardium, before finally washing out (Fig. 1.31). In order to acquire images quickly, DCE-MRI perfusion imaging is generally performed as a single-shot technique with a fast (or turbo) spoiled gradient echo (FGE), balanced steady-state free precession (bSSFP) or echo-planar imaging (EPI) pulse sequence (Fig. 1.32). All three sequences are fast, having a very short TR. Usually 3–4 short-axis views of the ventricle are acquired to assess the perfusion at basal, middle-cavity and apex level during breath-hold.

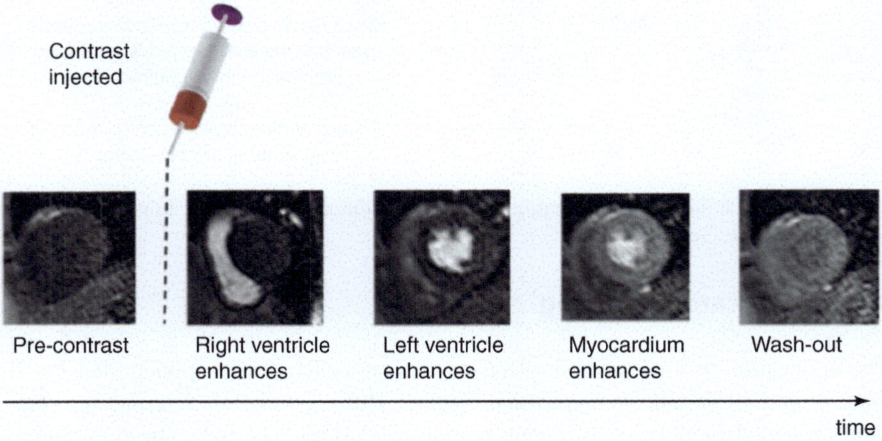

Fig. 1.31 Contrast agent is injected intravenously and can be seen as signal enhancement in the right ventricular cavity (RV) followed by the left ventricular cavity (LV) and more gradually in the myocardium, before finally washing out (from J Cardiovasc Magn Reson. 2012 Sep 20;14:66)

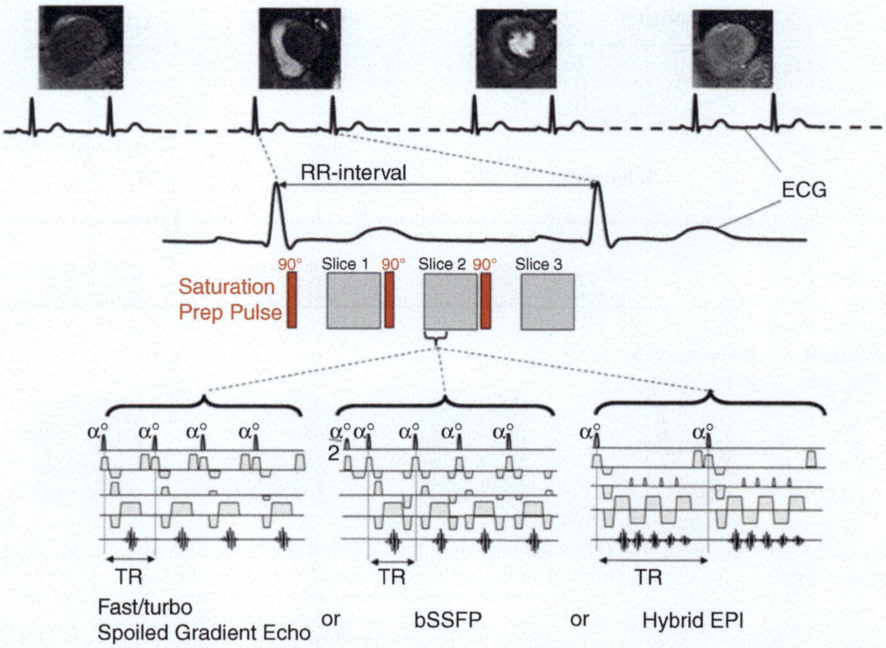

Fig. 1.32 In order to acquire images quickly, DCE-MRI perfusion imaging is generally performed as a single-shot technique with a fast (or turbo) spoiled gradient echo (FGE), balanced steady-state free precession (bSSFP) or echo planar imaging (EPI) pulse sequence (from J Cardiovasc Magn Reson. 2012 Sep 20;14:66)

DCE-MR images should be T1-weighted in order to maximize the effect of the contrast agent on signal intensity. For this reason perfusion imaging is usually carried out using a saturation recovery preparation pulse (Fig. 1.32). T1 weighting is controlled by careful selection of the saturation time (TS). Typically each imaging slice is preceded by a preparation pulse so that there are as many preparation pulses as there are slices in a given RR interval. A typical TS for cardiac perfusion imaging is around 100 ms.

Image degradation by cardiac motion is dealt with, as far as possible, by limiting the image data acquisition window, so the use of ECG triggering serves only to determine at what phase of the cardiac cycle the heart will be imaged. This is set by the trigger delay (TD), which is the time from the ECG R wave to the time of the acquisition of the central line of k-space (Fig. 1.33).

Endocardial perfusion defects may occur at any point in the left ventricular wall, and so maximizing the coverage of the left ventricle is important. The AHA recommends that three short-axis slices are acquired to cover basal, mid and apical regions of the left ventricle and that a spatial resolution of at least 2.5 mm is necessary to be able to reliably detect subendocardial defects. The most common method of reporting myocardial perfusion is by visual analysis of the dynamic series: regions that

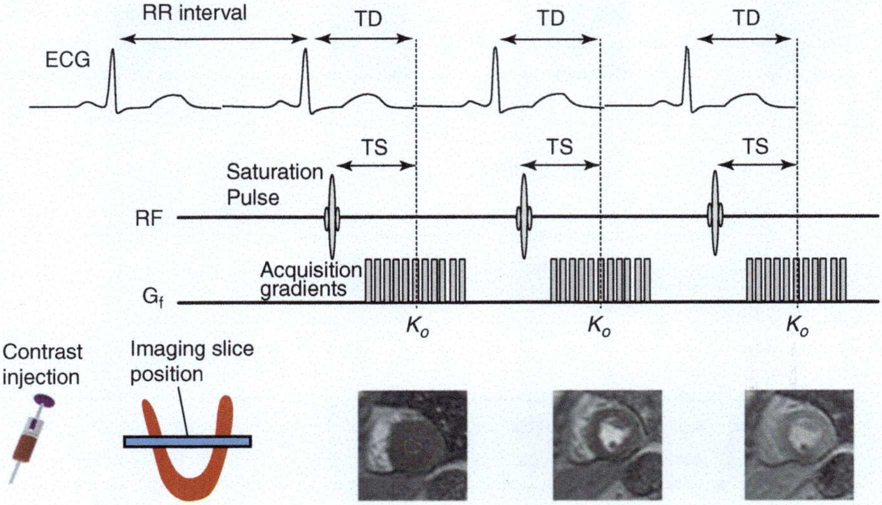

Fig. 1.33 The trigger delay (TD) is the time from the ECG R wave to the time of the acquisition of the central line of k-space (from J Cardiovasc Magn Reson. 2012 Sep 20;14:66)

appear transiently as areas of relative reduced signal intensity are taken to be due to a physiologically significant reduction to myocardial blood flow and recorded as a "perfusion defect".

A common troublesome artefact that can occur with perfusion imaging is the so-called *dark rim artefact*. It is a transient signal void at the endocardial boundary and is easily mistaken for genuine subendocardial perfusion defects. Typical features of the artefact are that it lasts few heartbeats and bSSFP is more prone to this artefact. It has been related to motion, increased magnetic field distortions, etc.

1.7.6.2 Early and Late Gadolinium Enhancement (LGE)

These are simple and robust techniques that are widely used in CMR exams. They involve the intravenous administration of gadolinium-based contrast agents (0.1 to 0.2 mmol/kg of a gadolinium chelate) that shorten T1 time of tissues, and it is followed by the acquisition of T1-weighted images of the myocardium by an inversion recovery technique.

Early gadolinium enhancement (EGE) is searched soon after the injection of the contrast up to 5 min usually with the acquisition of the three main long-axis views (four chambers, two chambers and left ventricle outflow tract). Late gadolinium enhancement (LGE) images are acquired after 10 min from the injection.

The clinical applications include detection of thrombus in the left ventricle (EGE), detection of hyperaemia in the myocardium (EGE), presence of microvascular obstruction (MVO) as evidence of the no-reflow phenomenon (EGE), presence of assessment of myocardial viability (presence of fibrosis by LGE) and detection of non-ischemic fibrosis and scar within the myocardium (LGE).

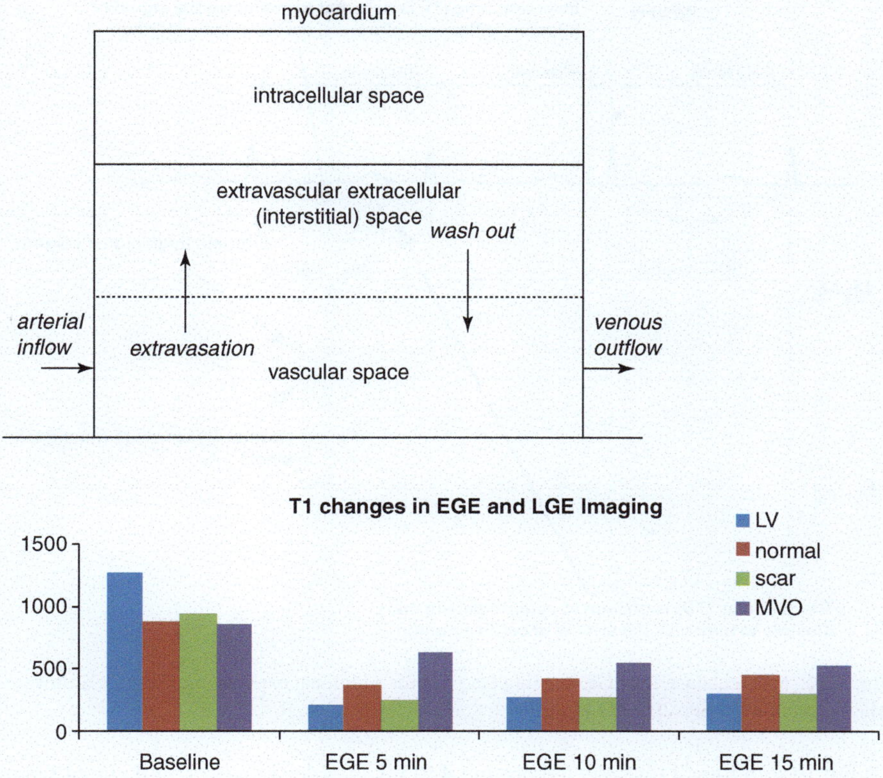

Fig. 1.34 Gadolinium contrast agent kinetics and T1 changes in baseline, EGE and LGE imaging according to the time from contrast injection (from J Cardiovasc Magn Reson. 2012 Sep 20;14:66)

When the gadolinium contrast agent is injected, the contrast reaches the myocardium extracellular space if well perfused and decreases T1 time. Thus in case of MVO, the contrast is not able to get the non-perfused myocardium. In EGE imaging <5 min, areas with MVO will have a decreased signal compared to surrounded perfused areas of the myocardium. From 5 to 15 min, the signal from normal myocardium decreases because of the wash-out of the contrast, while in areas with fibrosis, there is a slower extravasation followed by a delayed wash-out. For the purpose of LGE, it is important the choice of a correct inversion time in order to maximize the differences in signal contrast of the fibrotic myocardium compared with the normal myocardium (Fig. 1.34).

For the assessment of LGE, images are typically acquired using an inversion recovery, segmented, fast (or turbo) gradient-echo sequence (IR-FGE).

The sequence is based on an inversion RF pulse to provide a T1-weighted imaging, and an appropriate inversion time is selected to maximize the tissues differences (see Fig. 1.35).

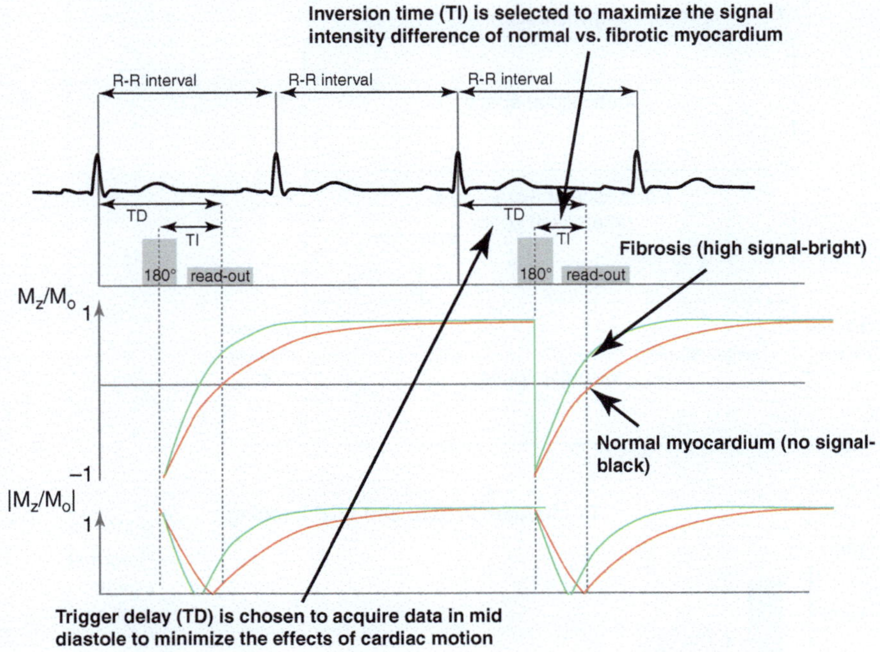

Fig. 1.35 MR sequence for LGE imaging (see text for additional explanation; from J Cardiovasc Magn Reson. 2012 Sep 20;14:66)

For EGE a long TI is selected around 440 ms in order to have a null signal from MVO tissue compared to normal myocardium, while for LGE the TI must be chosen with acquisition at 10 min after contrast injection to have a no signal from the normal myocardium (appears black) compared with the fibrotic myocardium (high signal and appears bright) (Fig. 1.36).

In order to find the appropriate time for TI, LGE imaging is preceded after the injection of the contrast by a T1 scout (that is a TI-sweep Look Locker module) to assess the best TI for subsequent LGE imaging. The TI changes over time and thus it must be empirically changed over time with the acquisition of images. For instance, in the example of Fig. 1.36, the TI is 300 ms at 10 min from injection but goes up to 320 ms at 15 min postinjection. The kinetics of the contrast is changing over time: normal tissue will have a regular wash-in and wash-out phase, while MVO and fibrotic areas will have a delayed wash-in and prolonged wash-out phase. Moreover for MVO areas, contrast can reach the MVO areas later due to diffusion from healthy tissue.

In the TI-sweep Look Locker module, TI values are changed incrementally before each image read-out. The resulting images display different contrasts and allow the operator to identify the TI which best minimizes the signal from normal myocardium.

To overcome the limitation of IR-FGE, where a wrong TI may affect the quality of images (e.g. bad quality of normal myocardium that appears grey instead of black

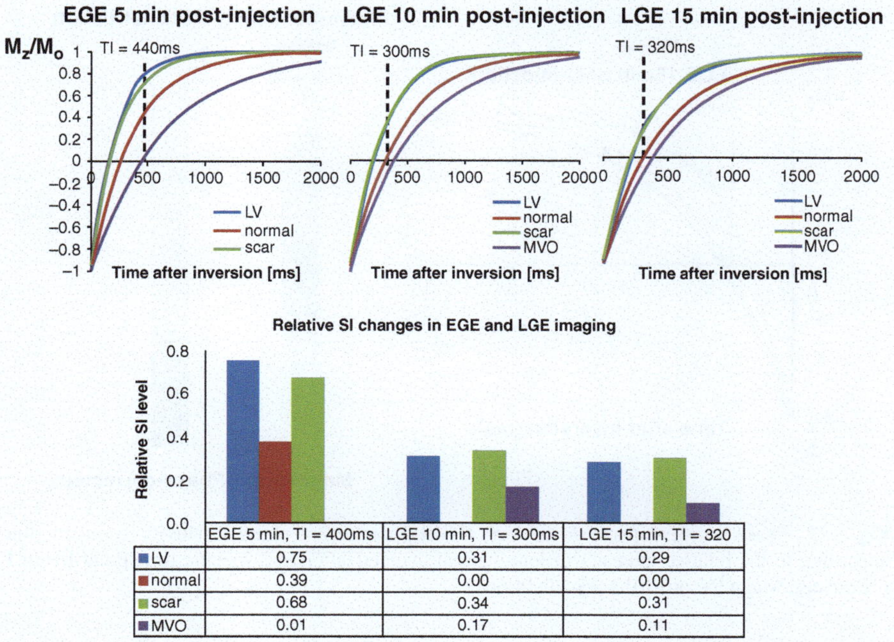

	EGE 5 min, TI = 400ms	LGE 10 min, TI = 300ms	LGE 15 min, TI = 320
LV	0.75	0.31	0.29
normal	0.39	0.00	0.00
scar	0.68	0.34	0.31
MVO	0.01	0.17	0.11

Fig. 1.36 EGE and LGE relative signal intensity (SI) changes according to acquisition time from contrast injection (from J Cardiovasc Magn Reson. 2012 Sep 20;14:66)

with a wrong choice of the TI), a new sequence has been developed: phase-sensitive inversion recovery (PSIR). In this sequence the acquisition is performed without the need to assess a precise TI since the relative values of longitudinal magnetization are evaluated and the signal intensity is reconstructed to create a scale of grey where the contrast difference between normal myocardium and scar is reconstructed according to the relative intensity of longitudinal magnetization at a specific time point (Fig. 1.37).

1.7.6.3 Magnetic Resonance Angiography (MRA)

There are three different approaches to get MR angiography: (1) *contrast-enhanced MR angiography* by using gadolinium-based contrast agents to depict the vessel lumen, (2) *non-contrast-enhanced MR angiography* to avoid the use of gadolinium-based contrast agents in patients with renal failure and (3) *respiratory navigator-gated coronary MR angiography* for the evaluation of coronary arteries (this technique prevents the effect of cardiac motion by ECG triggering to synchronize the acquisition in mid-diastole and prevents respiratory motion by special navigator RF pulses that allow the detection of diaphragm position to synchronize the acquisition with the respiratory cycle).

For all MR angiography methods, artefacts related to respiratory motion are prevented by breath-holding; this limits the acquisition time and the possible spatial resolution of the method.

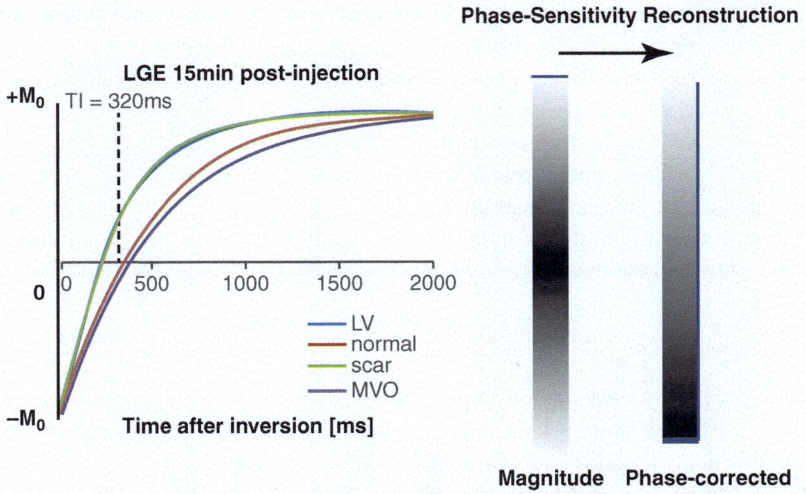

Fig. 1.37 Phase-sensitive inversion recovery (PSIR) imaging and phase sensitivity reconstruction according to the relative intensity of longitudinal magnetization at a specific time point (from J Cardiovasc Magn Reson. 2012 Sep 20;14:66)

Contrast-enhanced MR angiography (CE-MRA) is based on a spoiled gradient-echo pulse sequence (SPGR for GE, FFE for Philips, FLASH for Siemens) and the use of gadolinium contrast agent. The use of a gradient-echo sequence allows short TR times and fast acquisition; moreover it exhibits bright blood. CE-MRA is acquired using a 3D acquisition. A critical aspect of CE-MRA is the timing of the acquisition start after contrast injection. Images must be acquired at the time of the highest concentration in blood. The evaluation of the correct time can be achieved by two methods: (1) time delay measured by a small test bolus (that also allows to verify the patient circulation time and that the venous line is properly working) or (2) real-time monitoring of the contrast agent entering the region of interest using a dynamic acquisition (Fluoro-Triggered MRA by GE, BOLUSTRAL by Philips, CARE Bolus by Siemens), also named fluoroscopic triggering method (Fig. 1.38). In the last method, the starting of the MRA acquisition can be manual (the operator views bolus arrival) or automated if the MR system continuously monitors the signal intensity in the region of interest (ROI) in order to allow the automatic start of the acquisition when the signal exceeds a predetermined threshold.

The imaging of coronary arteries is one of the most challenging issues for CMR since coronary arteries are relatively small and motion artefacts from the heart and respiratory motion should be avoided. The most common sequence is a three-dimensional (3D) gradient-echo pulse sequence that provides a relatively enhanced signal from flowing blood with both cardiac trigger and respiratory gating. Data are acquired in mid-diastole to minimize artefact related to cardiac motion (Fig. 1.39a) and at end expiration with real-time monitoring of the diaphragm position using navigator echoes (Fig. 1.39b).

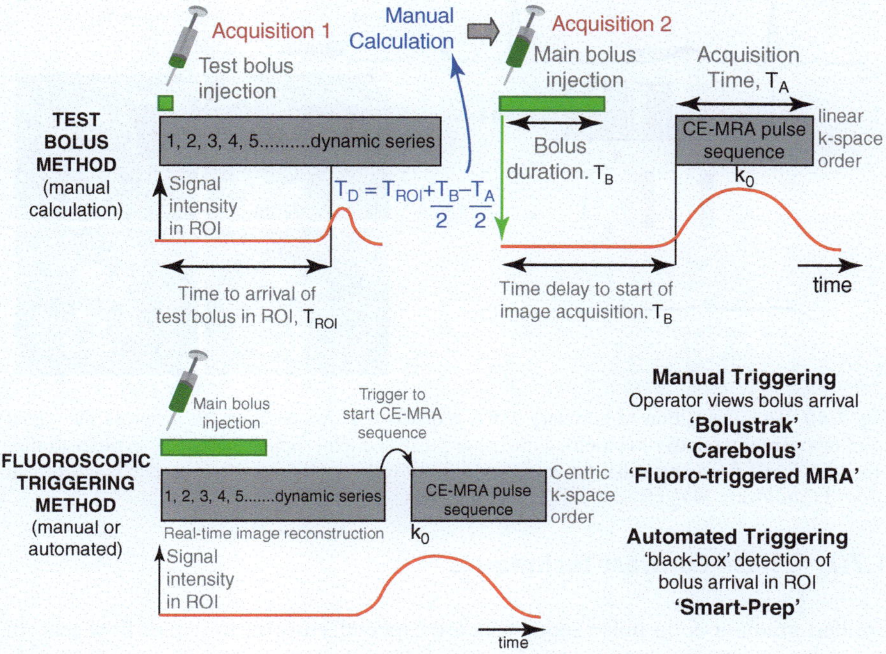

Fig. 1.38 Test bolus method vs. fluoroscopic triggering method (see text for explanation; (from J Cardiovasc Magn Reson. 2012 Sep 20;14:66)

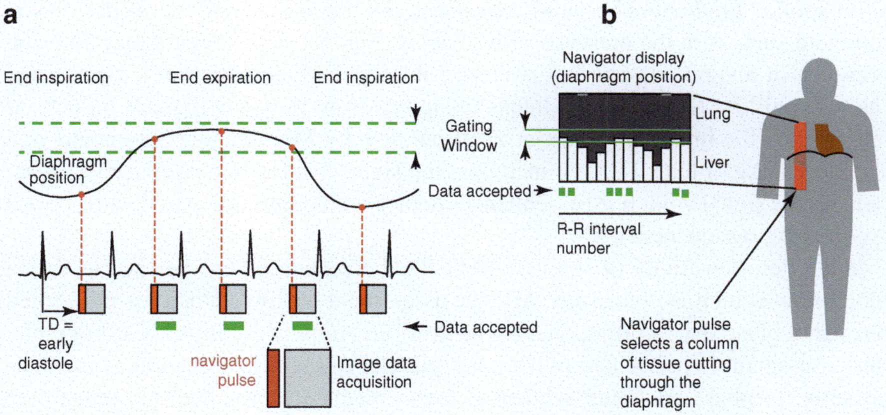

Fig. 1.39 Coronary MRA: (**a**) Data are acquired in mid-diastole to minimize artefact related to cardiac motion; (**b**) data are acquired at end expiration with real-time monitoring of the diaphragm position using navigator echoes (from J Cardiovasc Magn Reson. 2012 Sep 20;14:66)

The acquisition of coronary MRA requires a T2 preparation (to suppress the signal from myocardium relative to blood), a navigator pulse (Fig. 1.39) and a fat suppression pulse in order to suppress the signal from epicardial fat, and then 3D fast/turbo gradient-echo sequence is performed (Fig. 1.40).

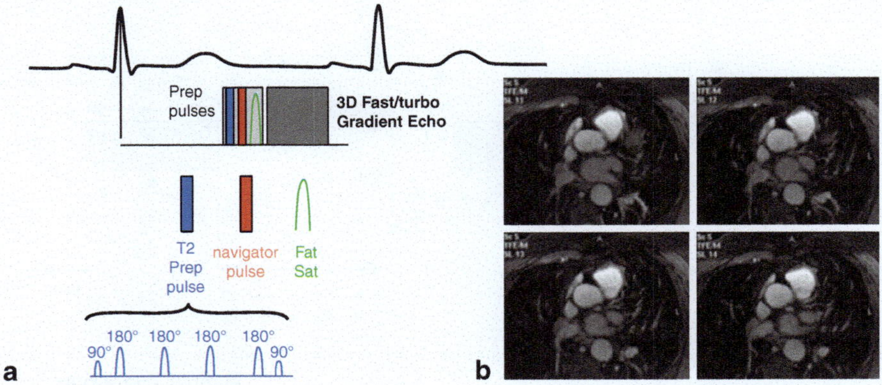

Fig. 1.40 The acquisition of coronary MRA requires a T2 preparation (to suppress the signal from myocardium relative to blood), a navigator pulse and a fat suppression pulse in order to suppress the signal from epicardial fat, and then 3D fast/turbo gradient-echo sequence is performed (from J Cardiovasc Magn Reson. 2012 Sep 20;14:66)

1.7.7 Phase Contrast Techniques

Spoiled gradient-echo pulse sequences are especially useful to depict flow jets. In these sequences the application of two equal but opposite magnetic gradients (G) after a specified time T is responsible for a change in phase of the moving blood that is proportional to the entity of the applied gradients, the time between the two opposite gradients and the blood velocity (v) (see Fig. 1.41).

In spoiled gradient-echo pulse sequences, the blood is bright, but if the flow is turbulent such as in the presence of a stenosis (Fig. 1.41) or a regurgitant flow, the presence of a signal de-phasing is responsible for the generation of a signal loss. Such signal loss results in low-intensity signals from flow jets that are influenced not only by the intensity of the jet itself but also by MR imaging parameters and sequences (e.g. a long TE time increases the signal void, while a reduced TE also reduces the signal void; bSSFP sequences depict smaller jets compared with spoiled gradient-echo sequences).

Such flow sensitivity of spoiled gradient-echo sequences can be used to depict blood flow velocities. In cardiac MR the assessment of flow velocity is performed through a plane that is orthogonal to the flow direction, while in echocardiography this assessment is performed by Doppler parallel to the flow direction as much as possible. In phase encoding sequences, two images are provided: (1) magnitude map and (2) phase map since MR signal is used to calculate both the signal magnitude (M) and the signal phase for each pixel (Fig. 1.42).

Phase maps changes related to magnetic field inhomogeneities (and not due to motion) are deleted by subtraction of phase maps to generate flow velocity maps.

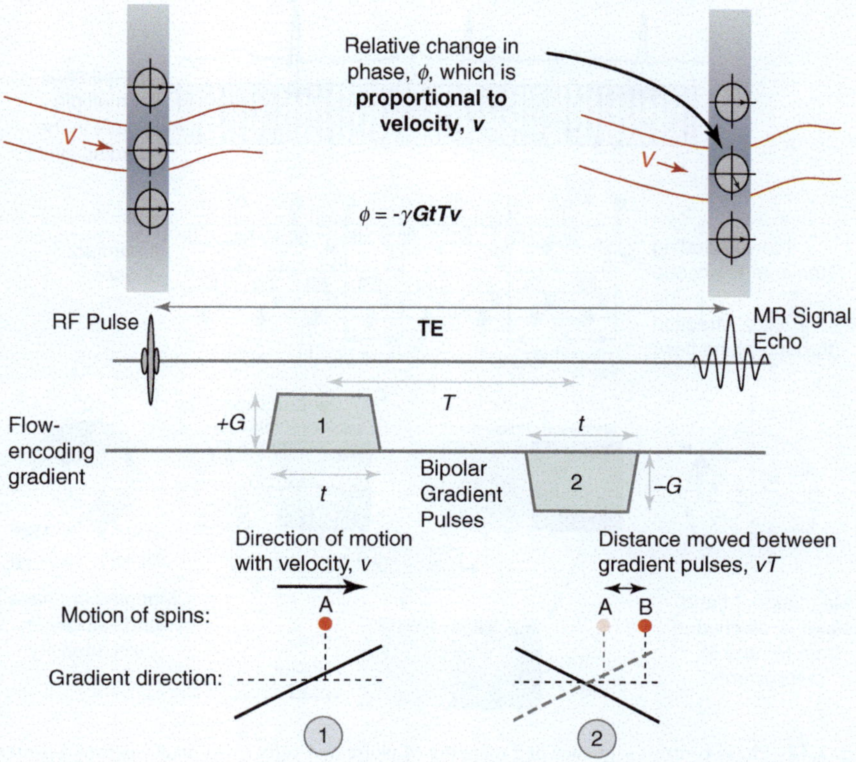

Fig. 1.41 Spoiled gradient-echo pulse sequences (blood is bright). See text for additional explanations (from J Cardiovasc Magn Reson. 2012 Sep 20;14:66)

The grey is set so that a stationary tissue appear as grey on the centre of the pixel scale. Positive or negative subtracted phase (corresponding to opposite flow directions) is mapped onto a higher or lower pixel intensity. Flow sensitivities are selected; a subtracted phase difference of 180° corresponds to the predefined maximum velocity or VENC (Fig. 1.42).

In these sequences the operator makes the choice of the maximum measurable velocity range (VENC). Such assessment can be based on operator estimation or also known estimated velocities by echocardiography. In the presence of encoded velocities that are higher than the VENC, the signal is interpreted as a negative phase shift and mapped on the lower pixel scale (black signal): this phenomenon is called aliasing and occurs if a low VENC value is selected by the operator (see Fig. 1.43 panel c, f in descending aorta, g in ascending aorta).

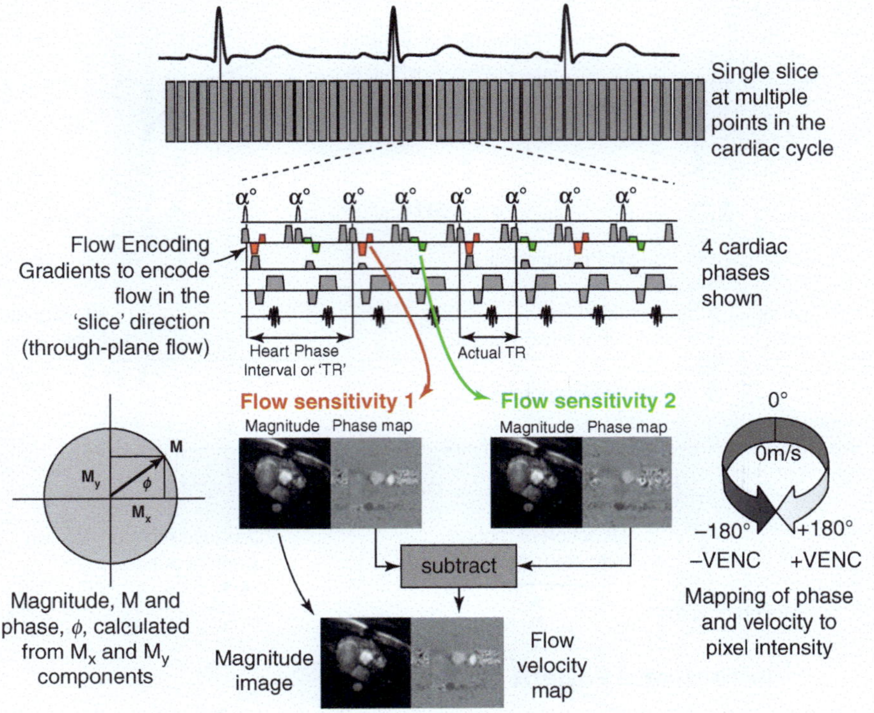

Fig. 1.42 Phase contrast sequence and mapping of phase and velocity to pixel intensity (see text for additional explanations) (from J Cardiovasc Magn Reson. 2012 Sep 20;14:66)

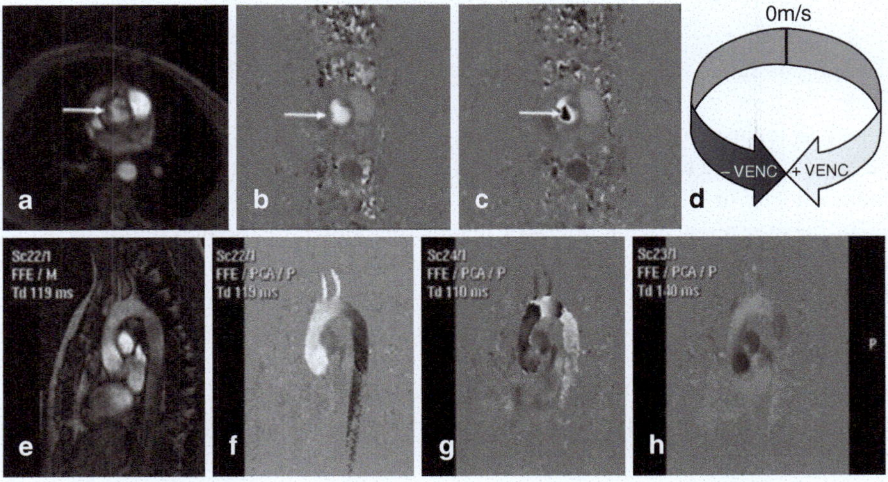

Fig. 1.43 Aliasing phenomenon in phase contrast sequences: in the presence of encoded velocities that are higher than the VENC, the signal is interpreted as a negative phase shift and mapped on the lower pixel scale (black signal): this phenomenon is called aliasing and occurs if a low VENC value is selected by the operator (see panels c, f in descending aorta and panel g in ascending aorta; from J Cardiovasc Magn Reson. 2012 Sep 20;14:66)

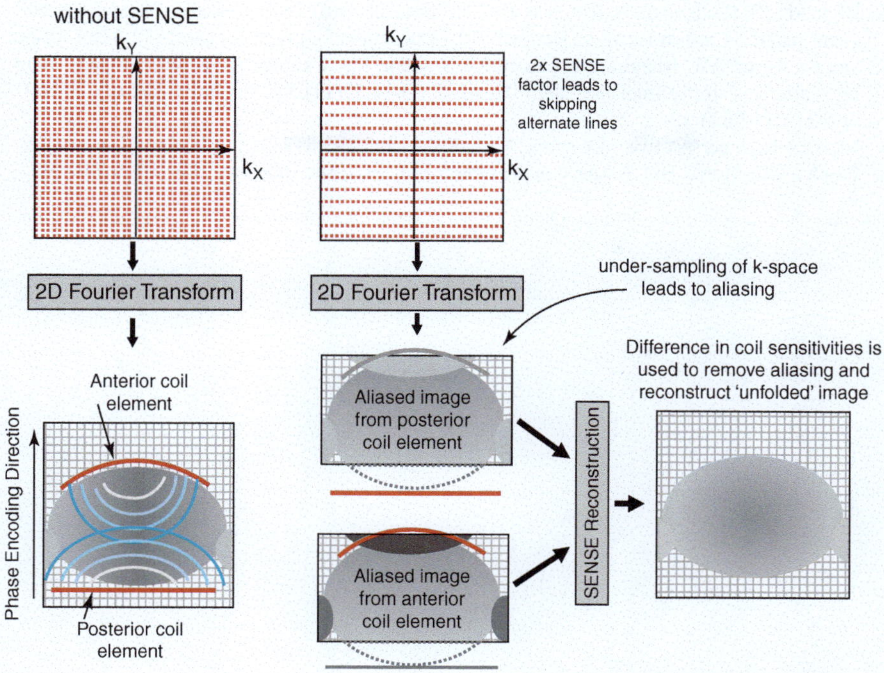

Fig. 1.44 Parallel imaging using the SENSE method (from J Cardiovasc Magn Reson. 2012 Sep 20;14:66)

1.8 Overview of Acceleration Techniques

Acceleration techniques are aimed at the reduction of the acquisition time through a reduction of the number of k-space lines. These techniques are complex and beyond the purpose of the present basic text. The most well-established technique is parallel imaging that is possible by the geometric distribution of coil array elements to restore the missing information coming from under-sampling of the k-space. Figure 1.44 shows an example of parallel imaging using the SENSE method.

References

1. Bruder O, Wagner A, Lombardi M, Schwitter J, van Rossum A, Pilz G, Nothnagelv D, Steen H, Petersen S, Nagel E, Prasad S, Schumm J, Greulich S, Cagnolo A, Monney P, Deluigi CC, Dill T, Frank H, Sabin G, Schneider S, Mahrholdt H. European Cardiovascular Magnetic Resonance (EuroCMR) registry – multi national results from 57 centers in 15 countries. J Cardiovasc Magn Reson. 2013;15:9. https://doi.org/10.1186/1532-429X-15-9.
2. Ridgway JP. Cardiovascular magnetic resonance physics for clinicians: part I. J Cardiovasc Magn Reson. 2010;12:71. https://doi.org/10.1186/1532-429X-12-71.

3. Biglands JD, Radjenovic A, Ridgway JP. Cardiovascular magnetic resonance physics for clinicians: part II. J Cardiovasc Magn Reson. 2012;14:66. https://doi.org/10.1186/1532-429X-14-66.
4. van der Graaf AW, Bhagirath P, Ghoerbien S, Götte MJ. Cardiac magnetic resonance imaging: artefacts for clinicians. Neth Heart J. 2014;22(12):542–9. https://doi.org/10.1007/s12471-014-0623-z.
5. Mezrich R. A perspective on k-space. Radiology. 1995;195:297–315.
6. Paschal CB, Morris HD. K-space in the clinic. J Magn Reson Imaging. 2004;19(2):145–59.

CMR Setup and Safety

2

Contents

2.1 CMR Setup

A CMR system is composed of three main electromagnetic components (Fig. 2.1):

1. A set of main magnetic coils
2. Three gradient coils
3. An integral radiofrequency transmitter coil

The main magnetic coils generate a strong, constant magnetic field. The strength of the main magnetic field (B0) is measured in tesla (T), being 1 tesla equal to 20,000 times the earth's magnetic field. Nominal field strengths range from 0.2 to 3.0 T for commercially produced clinical MR systems, with the most common field strength for cardiac imaging being 1.5 T (thus about 30,000 times the earth's magnetic field). Usually the main magnetic field is generated by superconducting magnets consisting of several circular magnet coils with many turns of wire (windings) carrying a high electrical current. The windings are made of a material that becomes superconducting when cooled to liquid helium temperatures (approx. 4 K or −269 °C). They are immersed in liquid helium contained within a vessel (the "cryostat") surrounded by two vacuum layers to reduce the boil-off rate of the liquid helium. The cryostat has a central bore open at both ends of the magnet (the patient bore). The patient is positioned within the central bore of the magnet (Fig. 2.1a). The magnet coils are positioned to generate a highly uniform magnetic field at the centre of the patient bore

M. Imazio et al., *Learning Cardiac Magnetic Resonance*,
https://doi.org/10.1007/978-3-030-11608-8_2

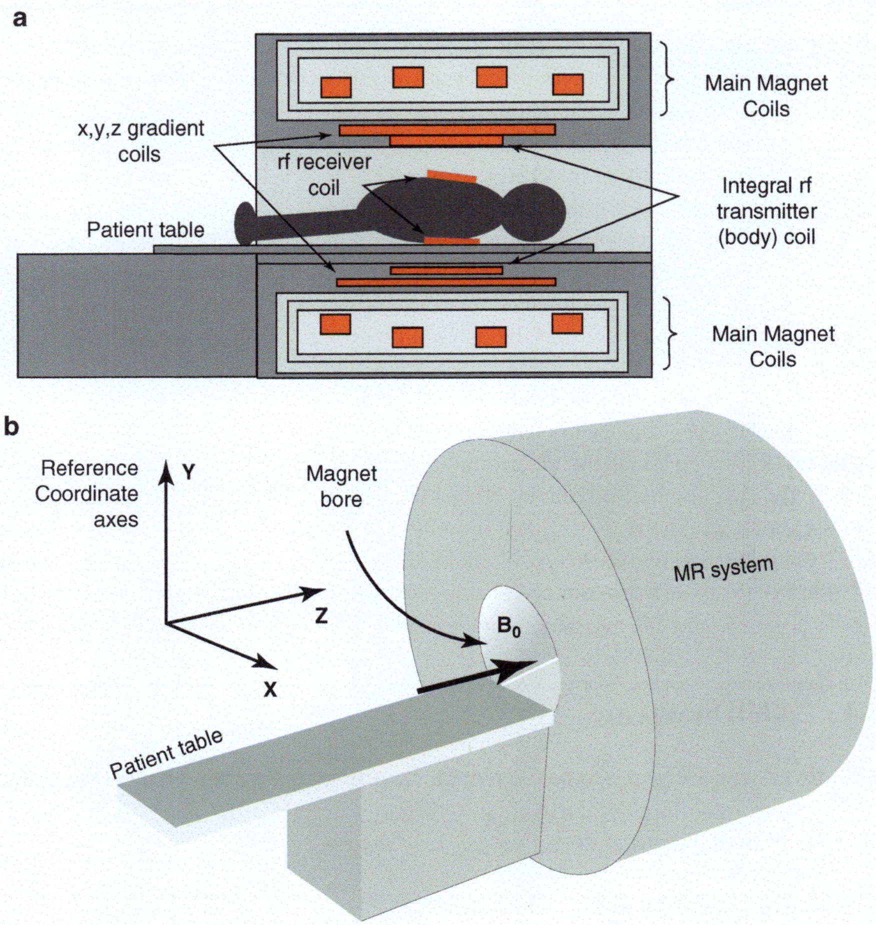

Fig. 2.1 The CMR scan (see text for explanation; from J Cardiovasc Magn Reson. 2010 Nov 30;12:71 open access)

typically over a spherical region between 45 and 50 cm in diameter, known as the homogeneous volume. The homogeneity of the magnetic field is maintained by passive shimming (at the installation of the magnet when small pieces of steel are placed around the inside of the magnet bore to modify the magnetic field so that it has the best uniformity) and active shimming by using small magnetic fields generated by additional electromagnetic coils to correct any remaining variations in the magnetic field (e.g. by gradient coils or dedicated shimming coils). Once the magnet has been activated, it is always on, and such a strong magnetic field is a constant potential hazard, and safety measures should apply (see later in the chapter).

The reference coordinate axes are named z (parallel to the direction of B0), x and y (see Fig. 2.1b).

The three gradient coils generate a gradient magnetic field that can be rapidly switched on and off and that is superimposed onto the B0 so that its strength varies along the direction of the applied gradient field allowing the localization of the signal and the selection of slices of interest to be studied. The strength of the gradient magnetic field is measured in millitesla per metre (mT/m). Gradient magnetic fields are switched rapidly within the main magnetic field (they can cause nerve stimulation of the patients). Such fast changes produce gradient coils vibration that are responsible for the familiar loud banging noise that is associated with CMR. Such noises warrant hearing protection for patients.

The radiofrequency transmitter coil is mounted inside the gradient coils and generates a radiofrequency magnetic field that is named B1 and allows stimulation of selected slices of the body to be examined. This radiofrequency oscillates at a characteristic frequency in the Megahertz range (Larmor frequency; see explanation later in the chapter), the exact value of which is determined by the nominal field strength of the main magnet. The resonant frequencies for the three most common field strengths for CMR are, respectively, 42.6 MHz for 1.0 T, 63.9 MHz for 1.5 T and 127.8 MHz for 3.0 T.

The radiofrequency at the Larmor frequency is able to excitate the tissue hydrogen nuclei that re-emit energy as RF signal when going back to the basal state.

Radiofrequencies have the potential to cause heating of body tissue. The rate of energy deposition is characterized by the specific absorption rate (SAR) with units watts per kilogramme of tissue (W/Kg) and is carefully monitored and controlled.

For cardiac imaging a separate receiver coil allows to maximize the signal coming from the heart [2]. The MR signal is small; the voltage induced in the receiver coil is typically measured in microvolts and so it is very sensitive to interferences.

The main manufacturers of CMR scans are:

- GE www.gehealthcare.com
- Philips www.medical.philips.com
- Siemens www.healthcare.siemens.com
- Toshiba www.toshibamedicalsystems.com

2.2 Safety Issues

Since RFs may affect the CMR signal, the magnet assembly and patient table are isolated by possible environmental RF interferences by a RF shield (Faraday cage).

The access to a CMR laboratory should be controlled with specific signs outside the entering door to the controlled area, where the patient wait and preparation room, control room and equipment room are included (Fig. 2.2). Access to the controlled area is restricted to authorized staff and screened patients. The main magnet and the patient table are inside the examination or magnet room (Fig. 2.2).

The access to the magnet room that is protected by a RF shield made of copper or aluminium sheet to avoid external RF interferences is also restricted: no ferromagnetic materials are admitted here to avoid the projectile effect towards the main magnet. Moreover the door of the magnet room should be closed during CMR examination. The main magnet is able to generate a strong magnetic field at its centre but also a magnetic fringe outside. On this basis the general public should be outside a 0.5 mT threshold to avoid possible interferences with pacemakers, and this area should be clearly defined. Access to the examination room is also controlled

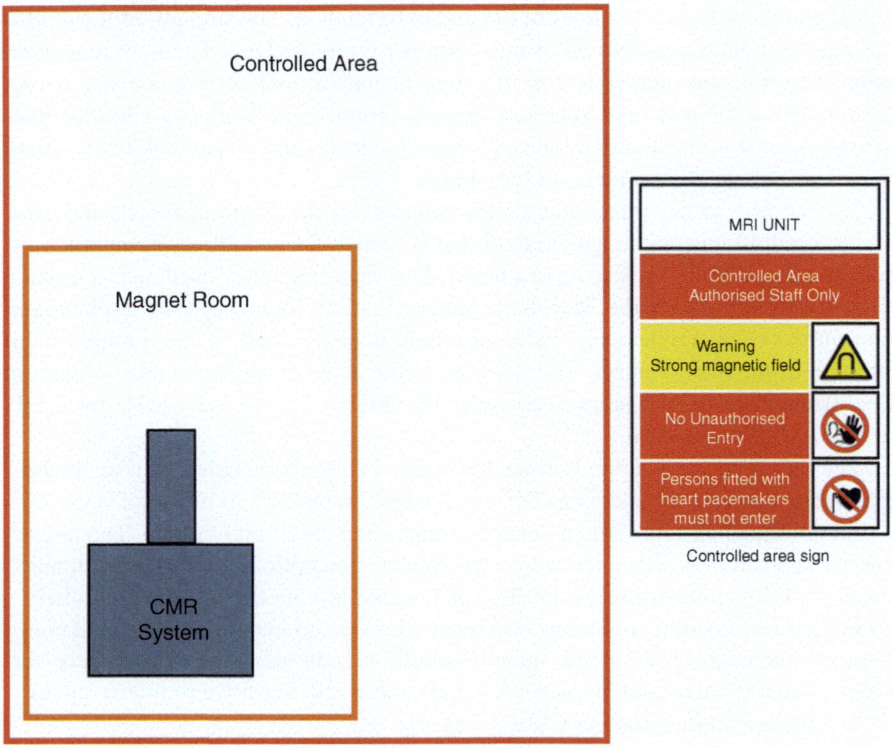

Fig. 2.2 MRI Unit: CMR System, magnet room and controlled area

and restricted in order to screen for the possible presence of ferromagnetic objects that may act as projectiles by attraction by the main magnet. The magnetic field damages items such as credit cards, mobile phones and watches. On this basis, such items should be carefully avoided in the magnet room.

Despite the presence of potential risks related to the presence of a constant strong magnetic field (the basal static magnetic field is about 30,000 times the earth's magnetic field in 1.5 T CMR systems), only few accidents have been reported especially related to pacemakers malfunction and some ferromagnetic objects projectile accidents. Safety is very important and the CMR laboratory is safe is the outlined precautions are followed.

2.2.1 Contraindications to CMR

Overall CMR is a safe examination if specific precautions are followed since strong magnetic field is maintained. At least 15 reports of mortal accidents due to MR scanning have been reported (mostly associated with use of pacemakers: ten with implanted PMs, two cases with an insulin pump, one case with a neurostimulator, one case with an aneurysm clip and one child killed by an oxygen cylinder due to a projectile effect). Additional severe incidents have been related to burns from wires and injuries due to ferromagnetic projectiles. Moreover fast switching magnetic gradients are responsible of generating loud noises up to 120 dB; thus ear protections are mandatory to prevent hearing losses.

On this basis a screening of the patient is mandatory in order to assess potential contraindications to MR scanning. Such screening is usually performed by a questionnaire (free questionnaires can be found and downloaded at www.mrisafety.com).

In order to understand the potential contraindications for MR scan, it is important to be aware of the potential risks of the CMR scanner (Table 2.1):

1. Missile effects and displacement of metallic objects in the body: the MR scan generates a strong constant magnetic field that attracts ferromagnetic objects that may become like missiles (ferromagnetic objects may be attracted with high speeds towards the main magnet); for the same reasons, metallic objects in the body can be moved and cause harm (this is especially important for the brain and the eye).
2. Gradient magnetic fields changes (noises and peripheral nerve stimulation).
3. Heating effects and interferences of radiofrequencies.

MR scanners typically produce noises when operating. Such noises are generated by the changing gradient magnetic fields. Such noises may reach 115 dB and over; thus hearing protection is mandatory for patients in order to prevent temporary and permanent hearing losses. Radiofrequencies (RF) are responsible of heating effects. Thus a maximum allowed absorbed energy per volume is monitored and named SAR = specific absorption rate. In normal operating mode, the whole body SAR is limited to 2 W/kg and head SAR is limited to 3.2 W/kg. In first level controlled mode, the whole body SAR is <4 W/kg.

Long wires and implants may be responsible of a strong local tissue heating (one accident was reported by local heating from an intracerebral electrode of a neurostimulator). An incident was reported with severe skin burns at both arms due to personal clothes with metal fibres in a Swiss patient (2010). On this basis it is important to avoid the skin contact with metallic objects and especially with

Table 2.1 Potential risks in CMR laboratory

Cause	Range	Potential risk
Main magnetic field (Always present)	0.5 to 3 tesla	Magnetic force and torque on ferromagnetic implants and objects
Gradient field (During image acquisition)	<80 mT/m <200 mT/m/ms	Loud noise Peripheral nerve stimulation Induced voltages in implants
Radiofrequencies	21–128 MHz (42 Mhz/T) <20 kW peak	RF-induced burns (extended implants, long wires and coils, large loops) Interference with active implants and devices
Contrast agent	Gadolinium-based	Allergic reactions (be careful to allergy to nickel, other metallic materials) Nephrogenic systemic fibrosis (NSF)

conducting materials with a loop geometry. Tattoos may warm up during MR exams since they contain conducting materials.

The most common contraindication for a MR scan is the presence of a non-MR compatible implanted device.

A specific labelling of items has been created to address the safety of objects in the magnet room by the American Society for Testing and Materials International in 2005 (Fig. 2.3):

1. MR Unsafe = Not safe in the magnet room
2. MR Conditional = Safe under specific conditions
3. MR Safe = Safe in the magnet room

If there is no label, the object should be assumed as unsafe.

Databases are available to assess the compatibility of the device (see www.mrisafety.com), and manufacturers also label their devices according to MR compatibility in reference manuals of their product.

A discussion on CMR scanning in patients with pacemakers and implanted defibrillators is reported later in Chap. 14.

In MR, common contrast agents are gadolinium-based contrast agents (GBCAs). Allergic reactions to GBCAs are rare (<0.2%); nevertheless a premedication is warranted in patients with known allergies, and a special attention also should be considered for those patients with allergies to metals (e.g. nickel).

A rare condition, named nephrogenic systemic fibrosis (NSF), has been recognized to be associated with use of gadolinium-based contrast agents. The first cases

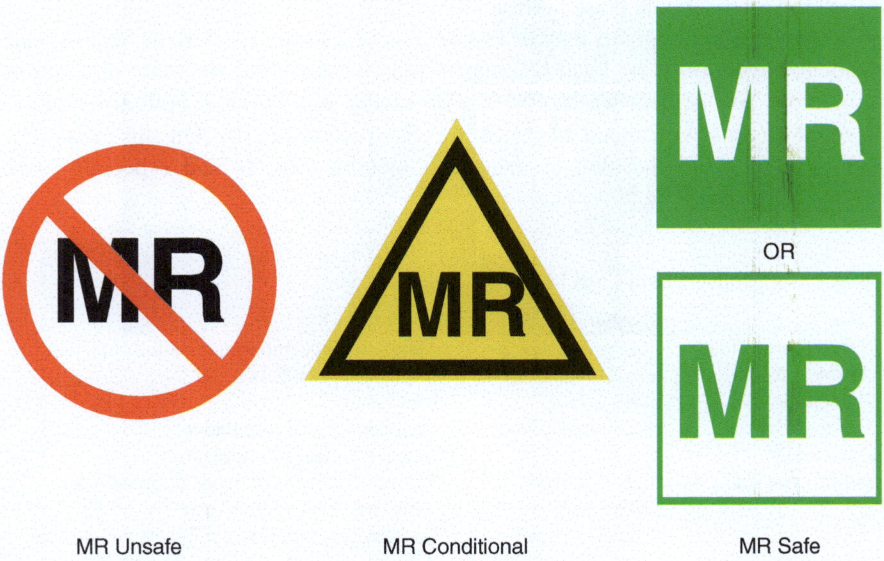

Fig. 2.3 MR safety labelling by the American Society for Testing and Materials International (see text for explanation)

have been described in 1997. The association between NSF and the administration of GBCAs has been proposed in 2006. The syndrome is characterized by the development of large areas of hardened skin with fibrotic nodules and plaques, and in more advanced cases, the disease may be progressive involving joints, eyes and internal organs. NSF develops over a period of days and weeks. In about 5% the course is rapidly progressive and severe.

NSF has been described only in patients with severe renal dysfunction (eGFR < 30 mL/min/1.73 m^2) or patients on haemodialysis. In suspected cases skin biopsy is warranted for the final diagnosis. No effective treatment is available. Fortunately no new cases have been reported after 2008 and the adoption of recommendations (see below).

The risk to develop the syndrome is considered to be related to the possibility of the contrast agent to release gadolinium, especially for linear chelates. Chelate structure and nature of bonding with gadolinium both impact agent stability. Ionic bonds have higher stability than do non-ionic bonds, and macrocyclic (ring structure) chelates are far more stable than those that are linear. Non-ionic linear agents have the lowest expected kinetic stability, followed by ionic linear, non-ionic macrocyclic and ionic-macrocyclic bonds. Of the 9 GBCAs commonly utilized clinically for diagnostic MRI, Omniscan and Optimark are non-ionic and linear, while Ablavar, Eovist, Magnevist and Multihance are ionic and linear. Gadovist and Prohance are non-ionic macrocyclic, and Dotarem is ionic and macrocyclic (Fig. 2.4).

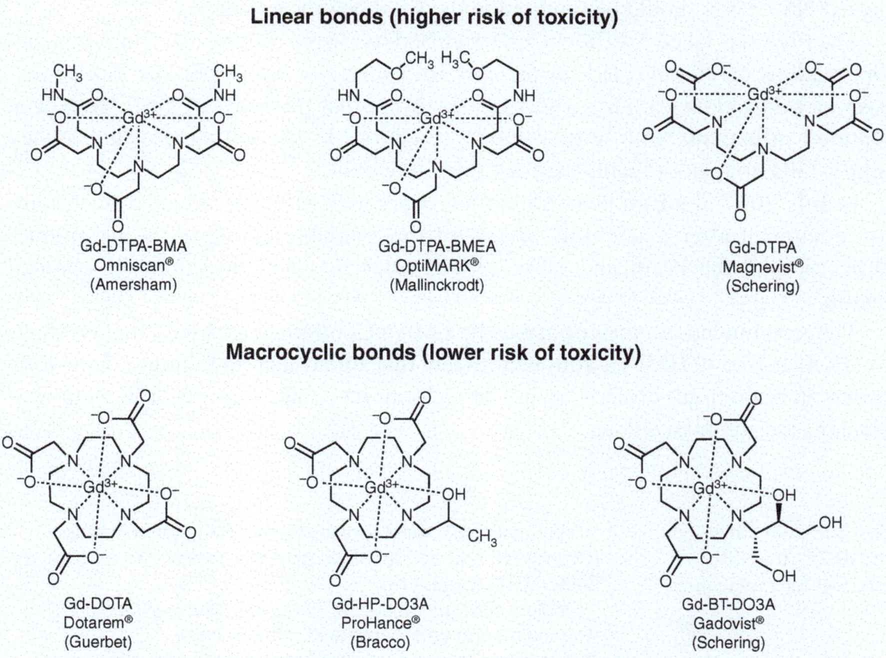

Fig. 2.4 Linear versus macrocyclic gadolinium chelates (see text for explanation)

The International Center for NSF Research (ICNSFR) has included 335 histologically confirmed cases. No cases have been reported in patients with normal renal function or chronic renal disease (CKD) stages 1–3.

The European Medicines Agency's (EMA) Committee for Medicinal Products in Human Use (CHMP) and the European Society for Urological Radiology (ESUR) have designated risk categories based on transmetalation theory in 2009 (Fig. 2.5).

The following recommendations apply (all patients should be screened for renal impairment):

1. *High-risk GBCAs*: they should be avoided with severe renal impairment (eGFR < 30 mL/min/1.73 m^2), patients around liver transplantation and babies <4 weeks with immature kidneys; use the minimum recommended dose in patients with moderate renal impairment (eGFR 31–59 mL/min/1.73 m^2) and children <1 year and wait 7 days between two MR scans with GBCA; breastfeeding should be stopped for at least 24 h.
2. *Intermediate-low-risk GBCAs*: warning for those with severe renal impairment (eGFR < 30 mL/min/1.73 m^2) and patients around liver transplantation; use the minimum recommended dose in patients with severe renal disease and children <1 year and wait 7 days between two MR scans with GBCA; breastfeeding may be stopped for at least 24 h.

Dosing and type of GBCA should be reported in the MR report. New or suspected NSF cases should be reported to the local healthcare agency.

The FDA has taken a different approach and has listed Magnevist, Omniscan and Optimark as contraindicated for patients with severe or worse chronic kidney disease or acute kidney injury. The FDA confirms that no cases of NSF have been reported in patients with normal kidney function. In the setting of acute kidney injury, GRF may not reliably assess kidney function.

In July 2017, the European Medicines Agency (EMA) has issued a final opinion document after a scientific review of the available evidence on gadolinium deposition in the brain and other tissues after repeated injections of contrast media.

The recommendations – confirmed by EMA's Committee for Medicinal Products for Human Use (CHMP) – follow a review that found that gadolinium deposition occurs in brain tissues following use of gadolinium contrast agents. The main conclusions are summarized as:

Fig. 2.5 Risk categories of GBCAs for NSF (see text for explanation)

***High risk: gadoversetamide (OptiMARK), gadodiamide (Omniscan) and gadopentetic acid (Magnevist, Magnegita, and Gado-MRT-ratiopharm);
**Medium risk: gadofosveset (Vasovist), gadoxetic acid (Primovist) and gadobenic acid (MultiHance);
*Low risk: gadoteric acid (Dotarem), gadoteridol (ProHance) and gadobutrol (Gadovist)

- There is currently no evidence that gadolinium deposition in the brain has caused any harm to patients.
- EMA has recommended restrictions for some intravenous linear agents in order to prevent any risks that could potentially be associated with gadolinium brain deposition.
- The intravenous linear agents gadoxetic acid and gadobenic acid can continue to be used for liver scans because they are taken up in the liver and meet an important diagnostic need. In addition, gadopentetic acid given intra-articularly (into the joint) can continue to be used for joint scans because the dose of gadolinium used for joint injections is very low.
- All other intravenous linear products (gadodiamide, gadopentetic acid and gadoversetamide) should be suspended in the EU.
- Another class of gadolinium agents known as macrocyclic agents (gadobutrol, gadoteric acid and gadoteridol) is more stable and has a lower propensity to release gadolinium than linear agents. These products can continue to be used in their current indications but in the lowest doses that enhance images sufficiently and only when unenhanced body scans are not suitable.

The specific recommendations for each contrast agent are summarized in Table 2.2.

In contrast, the US Food and Drug Administration (FDA) identifies no harmful effects to date with brain retention of gadolinium-based contrast agents for CMR, and its review is continuing but without restricting the use of any approved contrast media, including approved linear agents.

Common contraindications for CMR scanning are represented by:

- Old pacemakers and implantable defibrillations that are not MR conditional
- Metallic foreign body in the eye
- Deep brain stimulator
- Cerebral aneurysm clips
- Cochlear implant
- Magnetic dental implants
- Claustrophobia (up to 5% of patients)*
- Advanced renal failure and dialysis

Table 2.2 EMA recommendations for specific gadolinium-based contrast agents for RM according to the statement published in July 2017

Product	Formulation	Recommendation
Artirem/Dotarem (*gadoteric acid*)	Macrocyclic (i.v.)	Maintain
	Macrocyclic (intra-articular)	Maintain
Gadovist (*gadobutrol*)	Macrocyclic (i.v.)	Maintain
Magnevist (*gadopentetic acid*)	Linear (intra-articular)	Maintain
	Linear (i.v.)	Suspend
Multihance (*gadobenic acid*)	Linear (i.v.)	Restrict use to liver scans
Omniscan (*gadodiamide*)	Linear (i.v.)	Suspend
Optimark (*gadoversetamide*)	Linear (i.v.)	Suspend
Primovist (*gadoxetic acid*)	Linear (i.v.)	Maintain
Prohance (*gadoteridol*)	Macrocyclic (i.v.)	Maintain

Table 2.3 Absolute and relative contraindications to CMR

Absolute contraindications (no MR scanning) • Unknown active device, ferromagnetic implant or unknown aneurysm clips • Metallic fragment in the eye[a] or near-sensitive tissue (larger nerve or blood vessels) • Any implant known to be unsafe
Relative contraindications (MR scanning is possible after risk/benefit evaluation and written informed consent) • Active device not tested to be MR conditional (most pacemakers, ICDs, insulin pumps, neurostimulators, back pain stimulators) • Removable devices (e.g. hearing aids, pumps)[b] • Long wires or bars (>15 cm implies a risk of burns from RF), especially if near-RF body coil • Claustrophobia

[a]If unclear perform orbital x-ray
[b]Must be removed prior to entering the MR scanner room

Table 2.3 summarizes the current contraindications to CMR.

To summarize, when a patient is referred for a CMR exam, there are a number of safety issues:

- Rule out possible contraindications (ask questions on a prespecified questionnaire).
- The patients should remove all metallic issues before entering the CMR scan room (risk of projectile effect on ferromagnetic issues in the magnetic scan).
- Assess the renal function if gadolinium contrast is used (relative contraindication or precaution if severe renal impairment).
- Take an IV line.
- Use specific leads for monitoring.
- Use specific headphone or acoustic protection.

Each CMR may last from 20 to 40 min according to the indications and the adopted sequences. A defibrillator, all medications for emergency treatment and adequate expertise in basic and advanced life support must be available at the CMR laboratory at all times.

Key Points

- The main magnetic field is always on and requires precautions related to the capability to attract ferromagnetic objects.
- Patients should be screened for possible contraindications for CMR.
- Common devices that are absolute contraindications to CMR include most pacemakers (but MR conditional PMs are increasingly common and available), implanted defibrillators (MR conditional ICDs are increasingly available), insulin pumps and metal foreign bodies in the eye.
- Common devices that are not contraindications for CMR include most metallic heart valves, intracoronary stents, prosthetic joints, sternal wires, dentures and cardiac closure devices.
- In case of doubt regarding the possible safety of a device in a CMR environment, consult MRIsafety.com and device instructions manual.

References

1. Expert Panel on MR Safety, Kanal E, Barkovich AJ, Bell C, et al. ACR guidance document on MR safe practices: 2013. J Magn Reson Imaging. 2013;37:501–30.
2. ASTM Standard F2503–13. Standard practice for marking medical devices and other items for safety in magnetic resonance environments. ASTM International, West Conshohocken, PA. 2013. https://doi.org/10.1520/F2503., www.astm.org.
3. MHRA safety guidelines for magnetic resonance imaging equipment in clinical use. https://www.gov.uk/government/publications/safety-guidelinesfor-magnetic-resonance-imaging-equipment-in-clinical-use.
4. MRI Safety.com. http://www.mrisafety.com/TheList_search.asp.
5. Schwitter J. CMR update 2012. Juerg Schwitter, Lausanne, Switzerland.
6. ACCF/ACR/AHA/NASCI/SCMR 2010 expert consensus document on cardiovascular magnetic resonance: a report of the American College of Cardiology Foundation Task Force on Expert Consensus Documents. J Am Coll Cardiol. 2010;55:2614–62.
7. Levine GN, Gomes AS, Arai AE, et al. Safety of magnetic resonance imaging in patients with cardiovascular devices: an American Heart Association scientific statement from the Committee on Diagnostic and Interventional Cardiac Catheterization, Council on Clinical Cardiology, and the Council on Cardiovascular Radiology and Intervention: endorsed by the American College of Cardiology Foundation, the North American Society for Cardiac Imaging, and the Society for Cardiovascular Magnetic Resonance. Circulation. 2007;116:2878–91.
8. Pennell DJ, Sechtem UP, Higgins CB, et al. Clinical indications for cardiovascular magnetic resonance (CMR): Consensus Panel report. Eur Heart J. 2004;25:1940–65.
9. Sawyer-Glover A, Shellock FG. Pre-MRI procedure screening: recommendations and safety considerations for biomedical implants and devices. J Magn Resonan Imag. 2000;12:510.
10. Plein S, Greenwood J, Ridgway J. Cardiovascular MR manual. Springer 2015.
11. EMA opinion and recommendations on the use of gadolinium contrast agents. http://www.ema.europa.eu/docs/en_GB/document_library/Referrals_document/gadolinium_contrast_agents_31/Opinion_provided_by_Committee_for_Medicinal_Products_for_Human_Use/WC500231824.pdf.

CMR Methodology

3

Contents

3.1 Referral and Patient Preparation

A good referral is important for planning a CMR exam (Fig. 3.1). Additional readings for CMR methodology can be found in the reference list. [1–6]. It is important to address all the following items:

1. Patient demographics
2. Patient data (weight and height, pregnancy status, renal function, allergies, presence of arrhythmias)
3. Possible contraindications and detailed report of devices
4. The clinical indication to CMR and current available clinical and instrumental data

A good referral allows to identify patients that are unsuitable for CMR study (e.g. obese patients) or that may require specific preparations for CMR scan

M. Imazio et al., *Learning Cardiac Magnetic Resonance*,
https://doi.org/10.1007/978-3-030-11608-8_3

REFERRAL FORM FOR CARDIAC MAGNETIC RESONANCE

Patient Name

Date of Birth

Height

Weight

Renal function (Latest creatinine and eGFR)

Pacemaker/defibrillator, if yes specify:	Yes	No
Implants, if yes specify:	Yes	No
Metal in eyes (consider orbital x-ray if doubt)	Yes	No
Aneurysm clip/Brain surgery	Yes	No
Pregnancy	Yes	No
Asthma	Yes	No
Allergies, if yes specificy:	Yes	No
Previous reactions to MR contrast agents	Yes	No
Claustrophobia	Yes	No
Arrhytmias, if yec specificy:..	Yes	No

Clinical diagnosis

Relevant clinical and instrumental informations related to the diagnosis and CMR study

Specific clinical question/s for CMR study

Fig. 3.1 Essential elements for a referral form for CMR

(e.g. delay CMR study to achieve a better control of arrhythmias; consider scanning prone or sedation for patients with claustrophobia; device control and recheck after CMR scan for patients with pacemakers and defibrillators). Figure 3.1 summarizes essential elements for a good referral for a CMR study.

Patient preparation is based on the following steps:

1. Completion of the screening form to assess the final suitability for performing the CMR exam.
2. The patient is instructed on the modality of the MR exam (the presence of noise is normal, and breath-holding instructions are provided).
3. The patient is asked to change his/her clothes with hospital clothing in order to avoid the possible presence in the MR scan of any metallic object/material.
4. IV line is taken if contrast medium is necessary to complete the exam.
5. Placing of MR-compatible ECG electrodes on the patient's chest.
6. Placing of the phase array coil and a respiratory sensor on the chest of the patient.
7. A blood pressure cuff for blood monitoring is recommended in case of a stress study.
8. Headphones and earplugs are provided to offer hearing protection and facilitate communication during the MR exam.

Then the patient is carefully entered the magnet bore. Closing the eyes when entering the magnet bore may be a useful way to reduce the sensation of claustrophobia. The area of interest for the MR exam is placed in the isocentre of the magnet to ensure the maximal signal uniformity.

The CMR exam has to overcome several challenges: cardiac and respiratory motions and blood flows. A correct ECG monitoring is essential to acquire good images.

The ECG and a "good ECG signal" is essential for correct synchronization of MR data acquisition with the cardiac cycle. In current clinical MR practice, cardiac motion is dealt by using ECG gating/triggering techniques. Two techniques (Fig. 3.2) are used:

1. Prospective triggering is based on the acquisition of MR data after a prespecified ECG trigger (the R wave of the QRS) after a defined delay in order to acquire data at mid-diastole when the heart is relatively still in order to avoid cardiac motion effects on the quality of images.
2. Retrospective gating with continuous recording and retrospective sorting of cardiac phase without any loss of the last part of the cardiac cycle close to the R wave. It can be performed with small variations of the RR interval.

In patients with arrhythmias and consistent RR interval variations, although a possible correction of the variable RR time is possible by the option named *arrhythmia rejection*, there are two possibilities: (1) use of ECG triggering or (2) real-time acquisition at the expenses of temporal and spatial resolution.

The ECG signal is very important for a good cardiac synchronization. Careful skin preparation includes (1) removal of chest hair by shaving and (2) cleaning the skin.

In MR surface ECG electrodes are positioned close to each other on the left side of the upper torso as illustrated in Fig. 3.3. Usually a four-lead VCG signal is

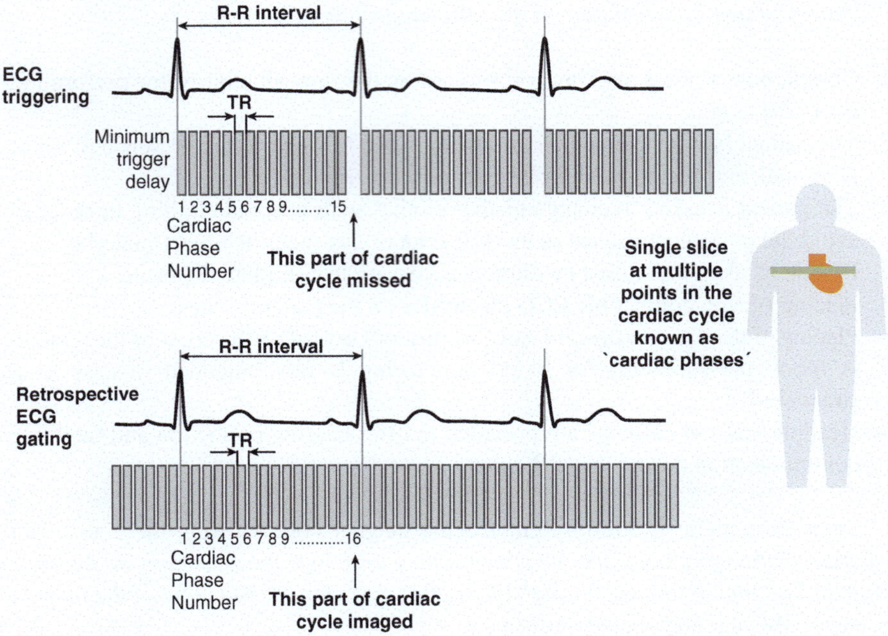

Fig. 3.2 ECG triggering and retrospective ECG gating (from Ridgway Journal of Cardiovascular Magnetic Resonance 2010, 12:71 (open access))

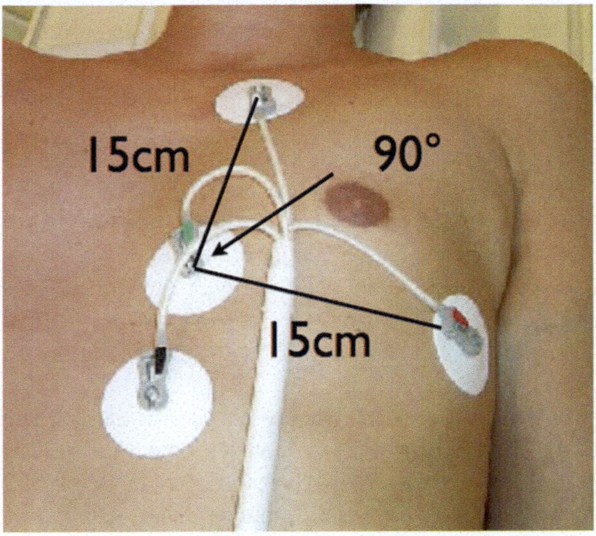

Fig. 3.3 ECG monitoring in the MR environment in a non-wireless triggering module (see text for additional explanations)

measured to reduce the effects of the static magnetic field on the ECG signal. Recommendations for electrode positioning vary depending on the available triggering module (non-wireless vs. wireless). Recommended lead positioning for the **non-wireless** triggering module is displayed in Fig. 3.3 and is set up according to these guidelines:

- White electrode at first intercostal space, just left of the sternum.
- Green electrode at the level of the xiphoid, just left of the sternum.
- Red electrode on the patient's left side, horizontally aligned with the green electrode.
- Black electrode in vicinity of green.
- White, red and green electrodes make 90-degree angle.
- Distance white-green ~ 15 cm.
- Distance red-green ~ 15 cm.

This placing offers to optimize the signal (avoiding placement too distant that may allow interferences for MR environment) and avoid loops that may favour heating and burns (the electrodes and cables should not act as an RF antenna). MR safe electrodes are used as well as high impedance ECG leads instead of conventional low impedance leads to minimize the risks. In addition the ECG cables are kept as short as possible, and fibre optic leads or wireless connections are used in modern system for signal transfer. For all these reasons, specific ECG electrodes and ECG cables provided by the MR vendor only should be used to avoid the risk of RF-induced burns.

All triggering-related parameters are derived from the heart rate that is entered. It is important to make sure that the entered heart rate matches the patient's actual heart rate.

An important alert for clinicians is to remember that the recorded ECG signal cannot be used for usual ECG evaluation since the ECG signal is affected and distorted by interferences of the electromagnetic field and by *magnetohydrodynamic effects*. The magnetohydrodynamic effects are induced by the blood flowing in vessels within the magnetic field. Since blood is a conductive fluid, a voltage is generated perpendicular to the magnetic field lines and blood flow directions. Such interferences are more pronounced during systole and may affect the morphology of the ST segment and T wave generating abnormal distortion of the ECG tracing.

3.2 CMR Protocols

The basic initial evaluation consists of localizer or scout scans to define the position of the heart in the thorax. Such evaluation is performed in the three standard orthogonal planes (sagittal, coronal and transverse) with low-resolution images.

3.2.1 Localizing Images and Planes

The initial acquisitions are based on low-resolution images that are acquired during free breathing and without ECG synchronization (so such images are prone to artefacts) in the three standard orthogonal planes (sagittal, coronal and transverse planes) using a spin-echo or gradient-echo technique. Such images are called **localizers or scout scans** (Fig. 3.4). Such images allow to confirm the correct positioning of the patient with the heart at the isocentre of the magnet, the RF receiver coil is correctly positioned and the appropriate array coils are turned on.

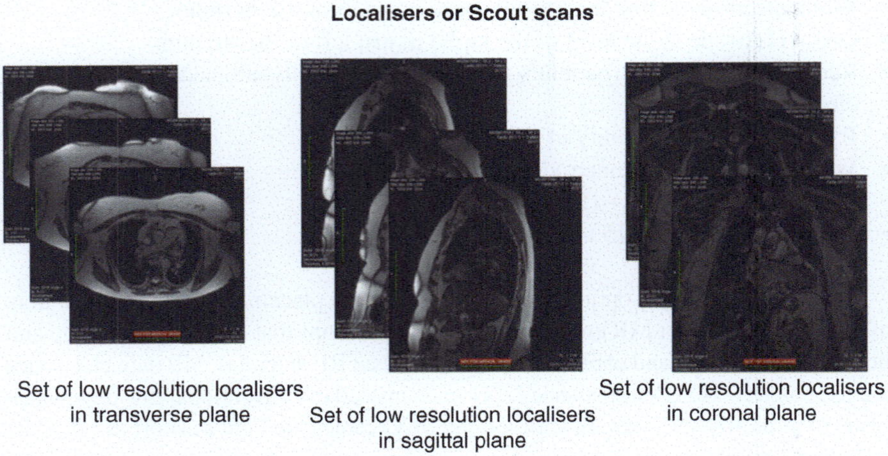

Fig. 3.4 Localizers or scout scans

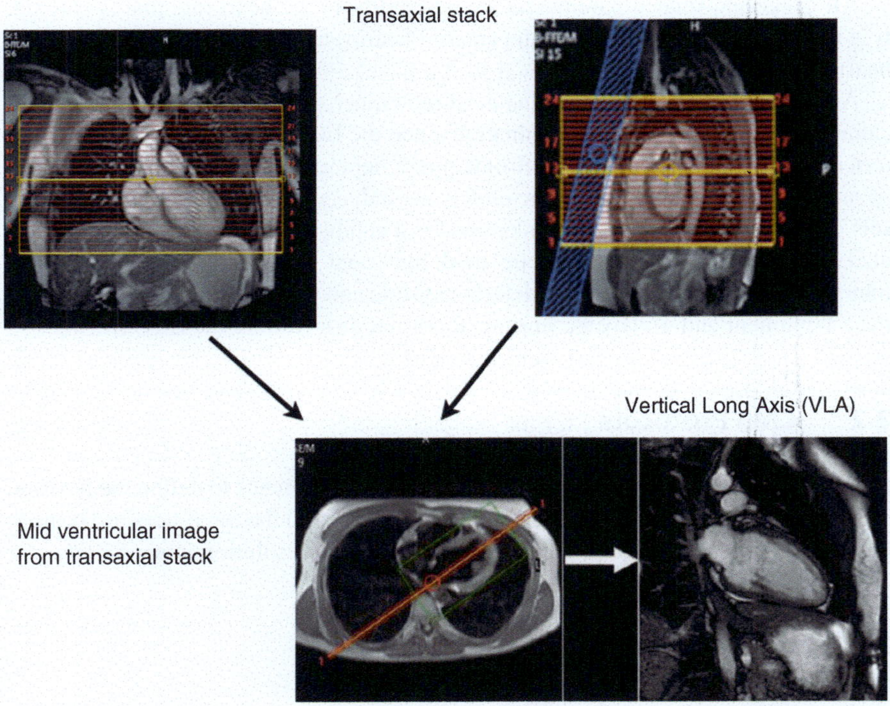

Fig. 3.5 Transaxial stack, mid-ventricular image from it and subsequent vertical long axis (VLA)

The second step is to acquire a transaxial spin-echo or gradient-echo low-resolution stack from the level of the diaphragm to above the aortic arch from the coronal and sagittal localizer images (Fig. 3.5). The resultant stack of transaxial images is used to obtain the main cardiac axes. From a mid-ventricular image that

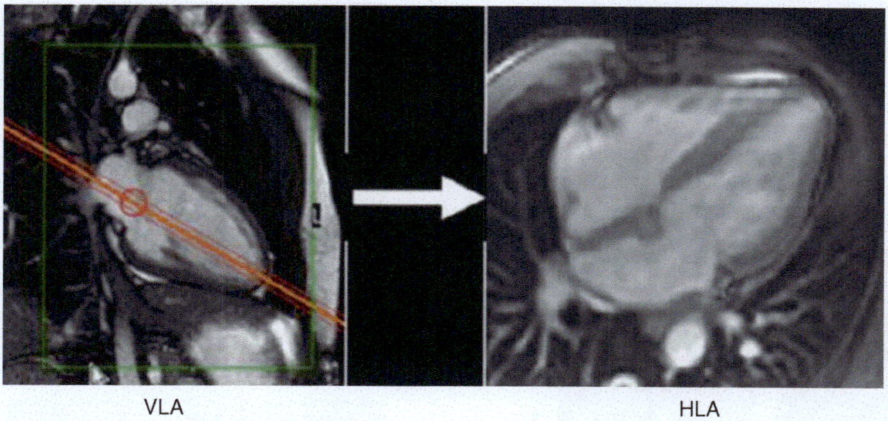

Fig. 3.6 VLA and horizontal long axis (HLA)

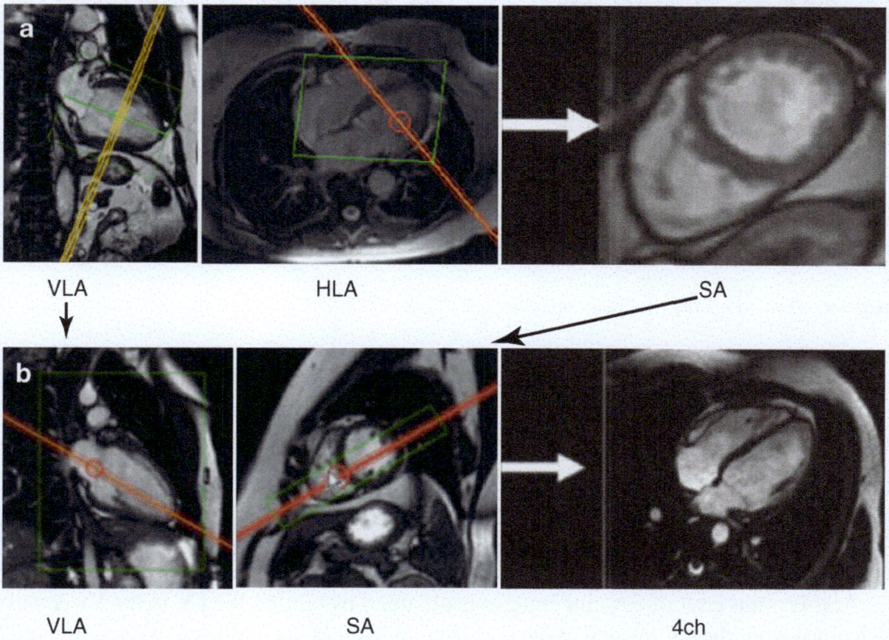

Fig. 3.7 How to get short-axis (SA) views of the ventricles (panel **a**) and true four-chamber view (4ch; panel **b**)

is cut by its long axis from base to apex, a vertical long-axis (VLA) cine is obtained (Fig. 3.5).

From the end-diastolic phase of the VLA, a section is conducted from the mitral valve to the apex in order to get a horizontal long-axis (HLA) cine image (Fig. 3.6).

Then we have to get a short-axis (SA) cine by cutting the VLA and HLA cines at the level of the mid-ventricular cavity parallel to the atrioventricular (AV) ring (Fig. 3.7a).

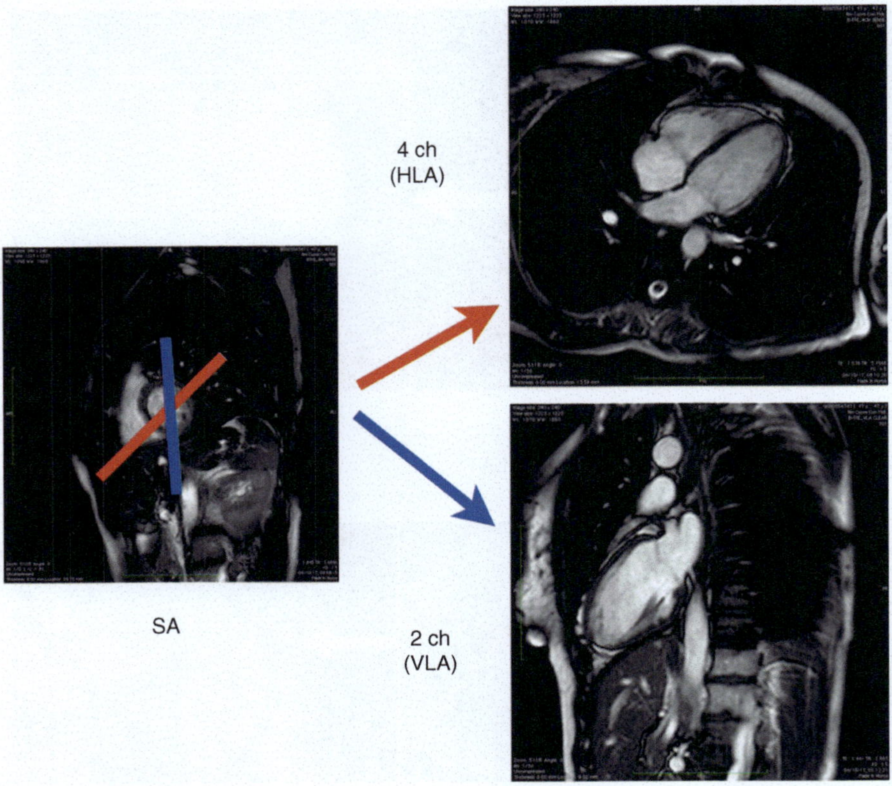

Fig. 3.8 How to get the true two-chamber (2ch) view

Then the 4ch cine (i.e. the four-chamber long-axis view of the heart) is obtained from two images by cutting the SA image at the level of the anterolateral wall and inferior interventricular septum and avoiding the left ventricular outflow tract (LVOT) and cutting the VLA along its long axis through the left ventricle (LV) apex (Fig. 3.7b).

The true 2ch cine can be obtained from two images by cutting the SA image at the level of the anterior wall and the inferior wall of the LV and cutting the HLA along its long axis through the left ventricle (LV) apex (Fig. 3.8).

At this point a set of SA cine images is obtained by cutting the LV in the VLA and 4ch cines from the AV groove to the apex (parallel slices are acquired to cover the full LV, typically with a 6-10 mm slice thickness and with a inter-slice gap 0-4mm to equal 10mm, and temporal resolution <45ms; see Fig. 3.9). SA cine images allow to perform a quantitative analysis of the LV and RV (volumes and masses).

LVOT cine can be obtained by cutting (Fig. 3.10a) the end-diastolic frame of the basal slice of the SA stack including the origin of the aorta: the cutting plane should be divided into two equal parts the aorta and LVOT. Such LVOT view is similar to the echocardiographic parasternal long-axis view. By cutting the LVOT cine by a plane that cuts into two equal parts, the aorta through the aortic valve is possible to obtain a 90° LVOT or LVOT coronal (see Fig. 3.10b).

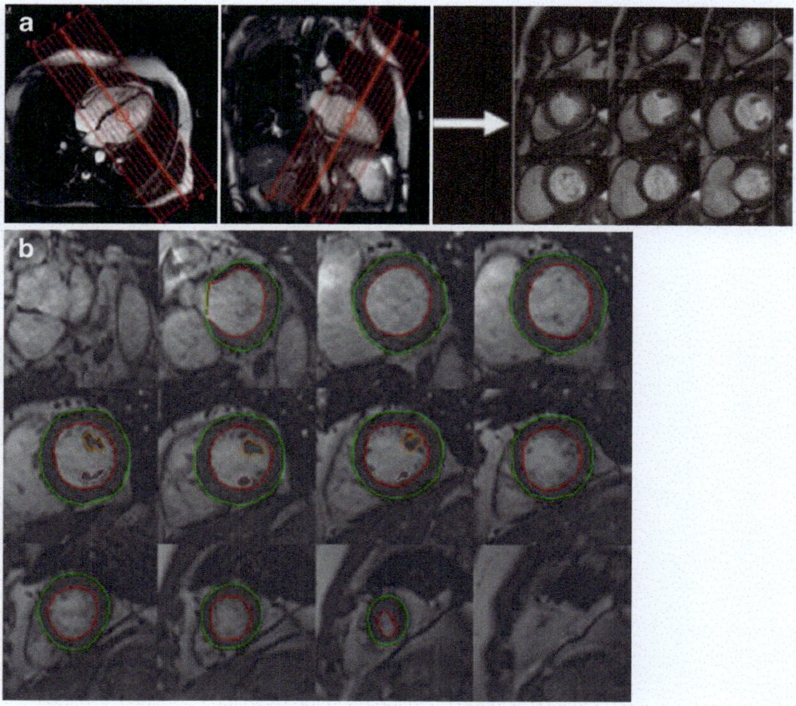

Fig. 3.9 SA images to allow quantifications of LV and RV volumes

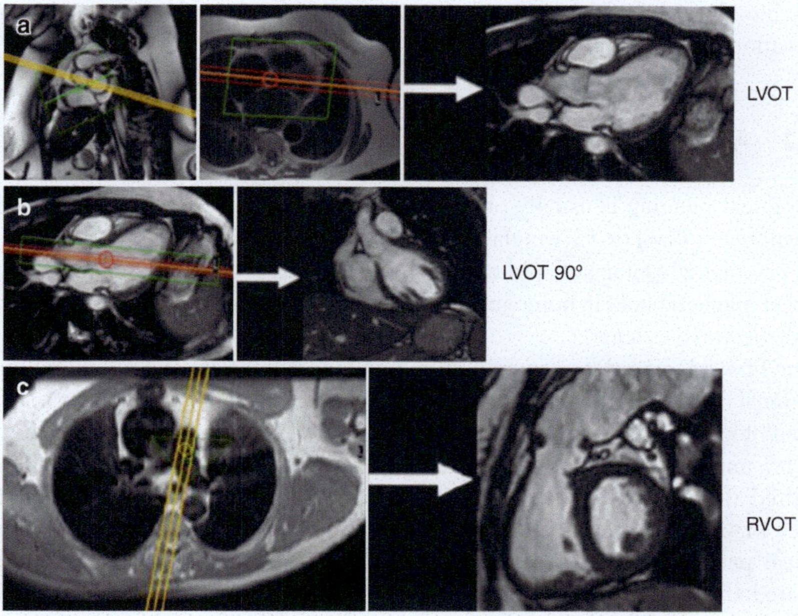

Fig. 3.10 How to get left ventricular outflow tract (LVOT) views (panels **a** and **b**) and right ventricular outflow tract (RVOT; panel **c**)

Fig. 3.11 Examples of T1-weighted images

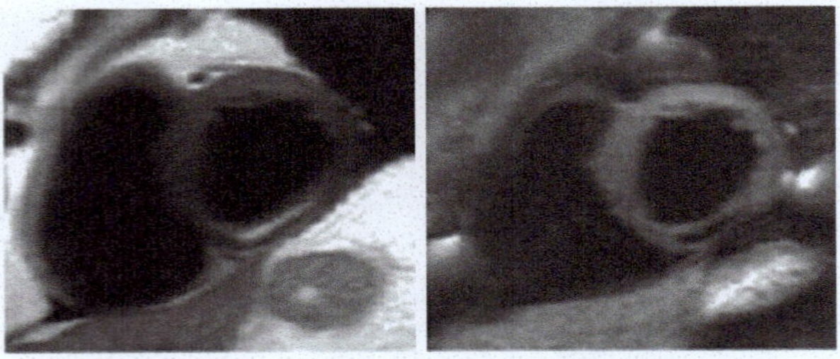

T1-weighted spin echo short axis images, with and without fat suppression

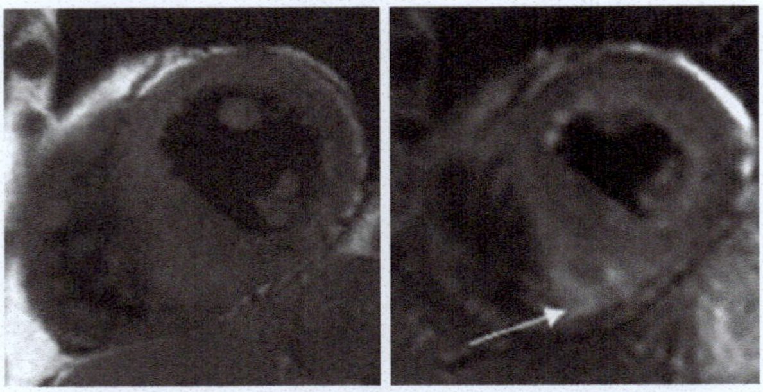

T1-weighted spin echo images pre-and post-contrast showing increased signal intensity in the 'mass lesion' in the inferior septum

In order to get the right ventricular outflow tract (RVOT), a transaxial T1-weighted black-blood stack is used cutting into two equal parts the pulmonary artery at its bifurcation (see Fig. 3.10c).

3.2.2 Anatomical and Morphological Imaging

Anatomical imaging is usually obtained by spin-echo pulse sequences that can be T1-weighted (T1w) or T2-weighted (T2w) to produce image contrast.

A peculiar advantage of spin-echo pulse is that these sequences are less affected by local magnetic field in homogeneities (e.g. they can be produced by sternal wires, prosthetic valves, stents).

On T1w imaging, fat appears with a high signal intensity (white), blood has a low signal intensity if flowing (black) and muscle has intermediate intensity between fat and blood (grey; see Fig. 3.11).

T1w images are usually performed 1 or 2 slices per breath-hold and can be acquired also with fat suppression in order to detect fat infiltration in the myocardium. T1w images can be acquired in any plane according to the studied anatomical part and are referred to as T1w black-blood imaging. T1w imaging is repeated after gadolinium injection. T1w images are ECG triggered and are still images that are obtained mid-way in the cardiac cycle and not in end diastole; thus it is not accurate to evaluate the size of vascular structures by such images.

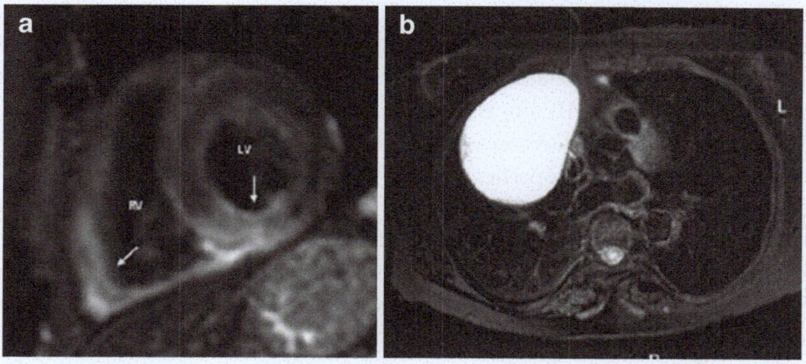

(a) T2-weighted triple inversion recovery short axis image demonstrating marked oedema in the inferior wall of the LV and RV.

(b) T2-weighted transaxial image demonstrating the very high signal intensity seen in a fluid-filled pericardial cyst.

Fig. 3.12 Examples of T2-weighted images

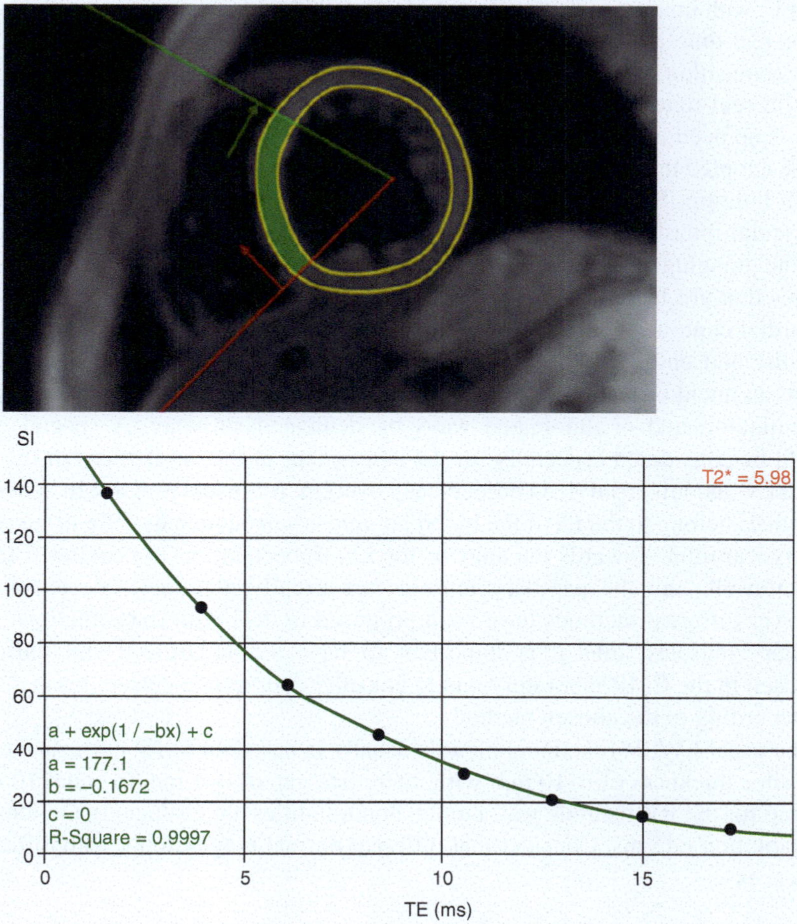

Fig. 3.13 Example of the assessment of myocardial T2*

On T2w imaging, the structure with an increased content of water appears with a higher intensity (brighter; e.g. edema or fluid-filled cysts are seen as white; see also Fig. 3.12). T2w images should be obtained before gadolinium contrast injection. Slice thickness of at least 10 mm is required to achieve a good SNR.

T2* relaxometry is used to assess the accumulation of iron in the heart and liver. Due to its ferromagnetic properties, the T2* time is pathologically reduced in the presence of iron. The T2* decay constant is obtained by specific software (e.g. Thalassaemia Tools, CMRtools, Cardiovascular Imaging Solutions, London) applied on specific region of interest in the interventricular septum and liver from a single breath-hold spoiled gradient multi-echo T2* sequence or modified black-blood sequence with blood signal suppression using a double inversion recovery pulse (Fig. 3.13).

3.2.3 Cine Imaging

Cine imaging is obtained using turbo gradient-echo and balanced SSFP techniques (bSSFP) with image acquisition during breath-hold by ECG triggering or ECG gating or real-time imaging with sacrifice of both space and time resolution to get faster acquisition.

With real-time acquisition as faster versions of TGE and SSFP techniques, there is no need of ECG synchronization and breath-holding; thus this technique can be adopted in the presence of arrhythmias or patients not able to allow a good breath-holding. Specific application of the technique may be the evaluation of ventricular interdependence in constrictive pericarditis (see specific chapter).

Cine imaging usually by SSFP allows to obtain a sequence of short-axis images that are frozen in end diastole and end systole to draw endocardial and epicardial contours of the ventricles, thus allowing the quantification of the end-diastolic and end-systolic volumes, ventricular masses and ejection fractions. The assessment of endocardial and epicardial contours can be made manually or in semiautomated or automated ways by dedicated software. A special care should be considered especially for the assessment of the basal slices of the LV where LV and left atrial (LA) borders may overlap. It is usual practice to consider that slices belong to the LV if the blood volume is surrounded by 50% or more of LV myocardium. Towards the apex of the LV, trabeculations are excluded from the LV wall, and the papillary muscles are usually planimetered separately. However different methods have been proposed to deal with trabeculations and papillary muscles; thus it is important to have a standardized and uniform approach in the CMR laboratory and to consider appropriate correct normal values according to the chosen method.

The usual LV/RV functional module usually is based on SSFP pulse sequence with slice thickness of 6–10 mm with inter-slice gap of 0–4 mm to equal 10 mm (no gap for the RV if subtle wall motion abnormalities are evaluated) and temporal resolution <45 ms. Consider that different normal ranges apply with different sequences.

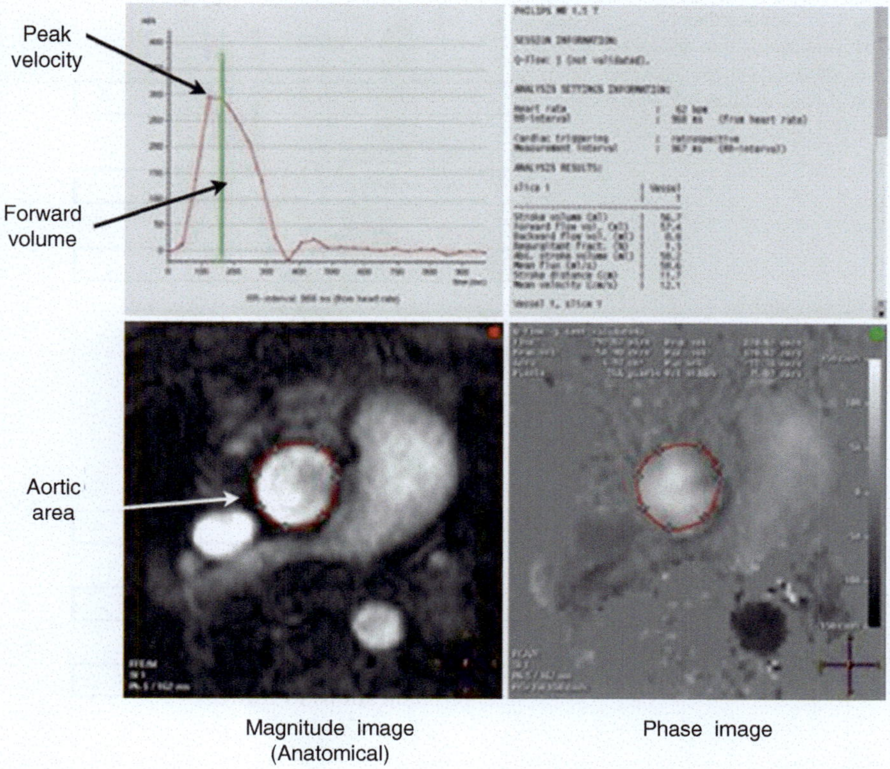

Fig. 3.14 Example of phase contrast velocity encoding technique to assess aortic flow

3.2.4 Phase Contrast Velocity Encoding

Phase contrast velocity encoding (VENC) techniques allow to estimate simultaneously the velocity at pixel locations and the area of the vessel of interest, thus leading to flow assessment. A phase contrast acquisition is based on two images: magnitude (anatomical) and phase (quantitative for flow with direction and velocity) images. The imaging plane is orthogonal to the expected flow (this is opposite to what happens in Doppler analysis of flows by echocardiography), and the correct direction of flow is selected.

An appropriate VENC must be chosen by the operator to avoid aliasing (usually VENC starts with 150 cm/s for normal systemic flow and 100 cm/s for right-sided flow, usually within 25% of the true velocity).

The acquisition is usually performed during free breathing and cardiac gating is retrospective. The vessel of interest is manually delineated at each phase of the cardiac cycle to correct for motion and size changes of the vessel during systole and diastole. Phase contrast images are analysed off-line using dedicated software that allow to estimate the peak flow velocity as well as forward and reverse volumes (Fig. 3.14).

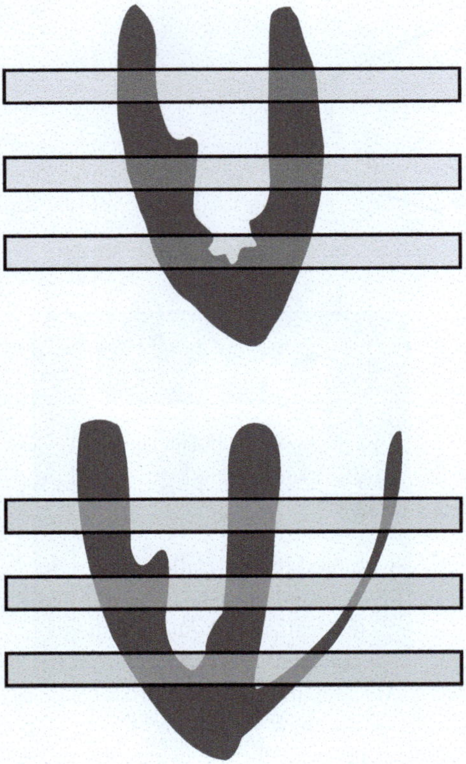

Fig. 3.15 Myocardial perfusion acquisition of three short-axis slices (apical, mid and base of the LV)

3.2.5 Myocardial Perfusion

The evaluation of myocardial blood flow by contrast-enhanced dynamic first-pass myocardial perfusion CMR is a routine clinical application (1) to detect reduced myocardial perfusion reserve in patients with suspected or known coronary artery disease and (2) for evaluation of cardiac and extracardiac perfusion of masses. Three imaging pulse sequences are adopted: (1) spoiled gradient echo, (2) balanced steady-state free precession (bSSFP) and (3) echo-planar imaging (EPI).

In myocardial perfusion study, at least 3 short-axis slices of the left ventricle are acquired (apical, mid and base of the LV) with a spatial resolution of less than 3 × 3 mm in order to minimize dark rim artefacts. In order to get reproducible short-axis slices, the rule of three of five slices is adopted. Considering a 4ch and 2ch view, the left ventricle is sectioned from base to apex by 5 slices that are 10 mm thick, and then good coverage of all the LV is achieved by increasing the gap between slices, and the central 3 slices are maintained (see Fig. 3.15).

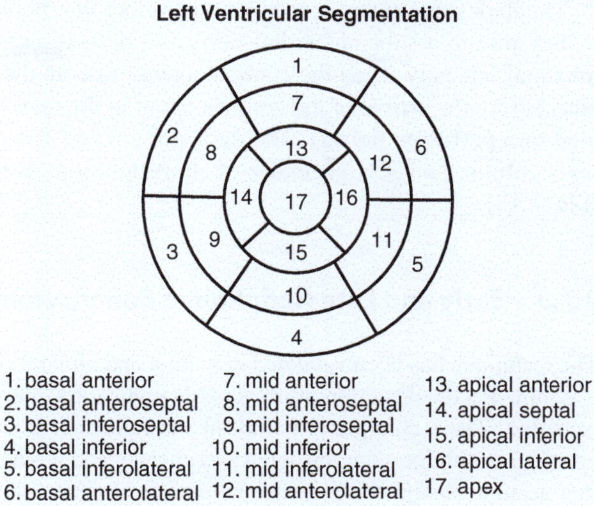

Fig. 3.16 LV segmentation according to the 17-segment model of the American Heart Association (AHA)

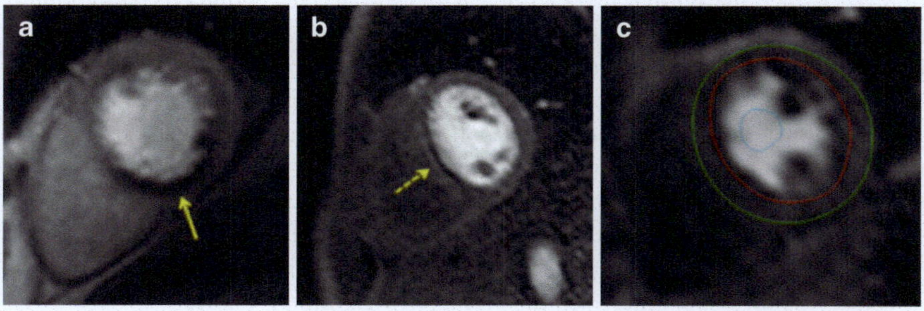

Fig. 3.17 Examples of perfusion defect and dark rim artefact. An inferior perfusion defect (panel **a**), a dark rim artefact (panel **b**; see text for explanation) and quantitative assessment of perfusion (panel **c**). From Schulz-Menger et al. Journal of Cardiovascular Magnetic Resonance 2013;15:35. Open Access

Contrast is given (0.05–0.1 mmol/kg at 3–7 mL/s followed by saline flush at 3–7 mL/s). Breath-hold starts during early phases of contrast infusion before contrast reaches the LV cavity.

The interpretation of the CMR perfusion images can be performed by visual assessment (if the coronary blood flow is normal, the myocardium has a homogenous grey appearance after first pass, while it is dark when a perfusion defect occurs; perfusion defect is localized according to the 17-segment model of the American Heart Association (Fig. 3.16) and compared with late gadolinium enhancement images to assess the presence of inducible ischemia, infarction, artefacts and normal perfusion) or semiquantitative or quantitative assessment by dedicated software (usually performed for research purposes and less common in clinical practice).

The dark rim artefact is a common artefact that is seen in perfusion sequences. It may mimic a subendocardial perfusion defect, and it is typically seen with a maximal intensity when the contrast agent peaks in the LV cavity (since this happens before the arrival of the contrast agent in the myocardium, it cannot be attributed to a perfusion defect). The dark rim artefact fades as the contrast enters the myocardium, and it is generally of short duration, usually 5–10 dynamic frames (Fig. 3.17).

3.2.6 Early and Late Gadolinium Enhancement

The technique has been validated in animal and clinical studies in the late 1990s, and it is aimed at the detection of irreversible myocardial damage either ischemic or non-ischemic. The technique is based on the injection of a gadolinium-based contrast agent. Gadolinium is administered as a chelate, and it is an extracellular contrast agent that accumulates in the presence of increased extracellular space (fibrosis, necrotic tissue with disrupted cell membranes that allow gadolinium to enter in the intracellular space) since the normal myocardium is densely packed with cells. Gadolinium shortens the T1 relaxation, and in this way, it is able to increase the signal on T1-weighted images. The contrast between normal myocardium and pathological tissue should be optimized by the choice of the inversion delay time to allow the normal myocardium to appear dark compared with the bright pathological tissue. For this assessment a "Look-Locker" or "T1 scout" sequence is run. This sequence is usually a 2D segmented inversion recovery (IR) gradient-echo sequence timed to read out the mid-diastole with a single slice acquired at mid-diastole. This sequence of images is conducted during breath-hold with a progressively longer inversion time. The operator selects the inversion time when the normal myocardium is darkest.

The protocol for the acquisition of early (EGE) and late gadolinium enhancement (LGE) includes:

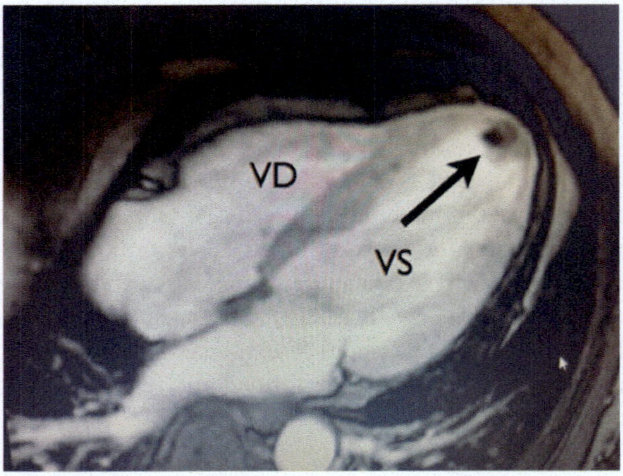

Fig. 3.18 LV thrombus detected by EGE as a "minus" (see text for explanation)

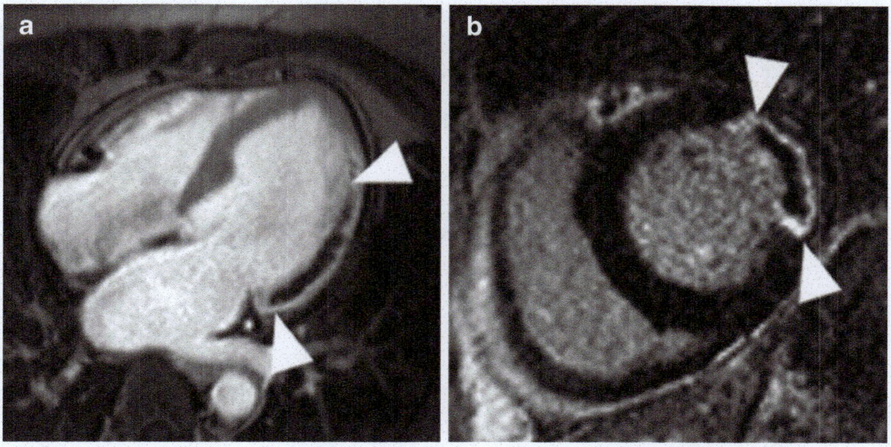

Fig. 3.19 Evidence of MVO (dark signal) within contrasted myocardium at the EGE image (panel **a**) and within the myocardial scar on LGE depicted as brighter area compared with the surrounding myocardium (panel **b**). Reproduced from Biglands et al. Journal of Cardiovascular Magnetic Resonance 2012;14:66. Open Access

1. Administration of a bolus IV of gadolinium contrast agent at the dose of 0.1–0.2 mmol/kg.
2. For EGE (essentially used for the detection of intracardiac thrombus and microvascular obstruction (MVO) in ischemic heart disease), imaging is performed immediately after contrast injection (no later than 5 min from the injection) with a fixed and long inversion time (TI) of 400–500 msec and long-axis views of the LV (4ch, 2ch and LVOT) are acquired. The normal myocardium appears grey, while intracardiac thrombus or MVO appears black (Fig. 3.18).
3. For LGE imaging starts around 10 min (shorter with lower doses) after contrast injection after assessment of the correct inversion time (TI) to optimize the contrast between normal and pathological tissue so that normal myocardium is dark and pathological tissue is bright ("white is dead") (Fig. 3.19). Usually a complete stack of short-axis slices of the ventricles is acquired, and then the inversion time (TI) is increased by 10–15 msec (since it increases with time) before the acquisition of long axis.
4. In-plane resolution is about 1.4–1.8 mm.
5. Read-out is usually every other beat but can be modified to every beat (if bradycardia) or every third beat (if tachycardia). In the presence of arrhythmias (e.g. atrial fibrillation), images are acquired every second or third beat.

3.2.7 T1 and T2 Mapping

The myocardium has its proper T1 and T2 relaxation time constants that can be affected by pathological processes. For the normal myocardium, the T1 is around 940–1000 msec at 1.5 T. T1 changes occur with diseases and may be affected also

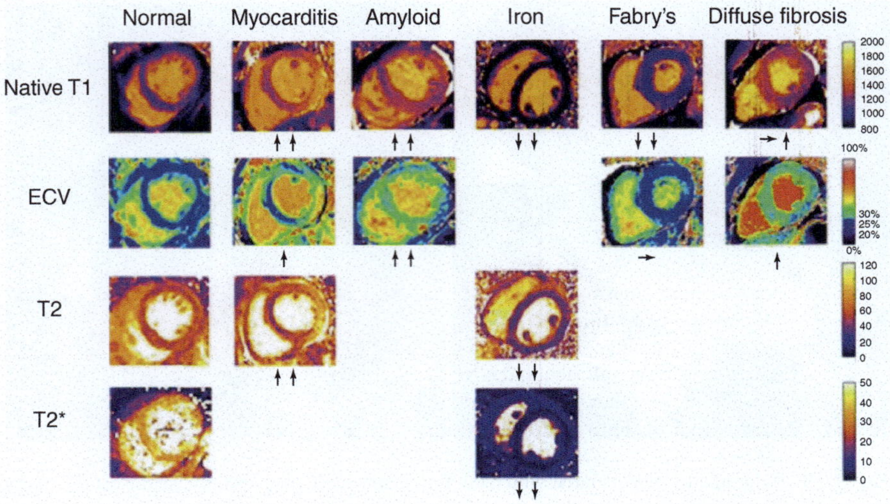

Fig. 3.20 Examples of T1, T2, T2* and ECV maps in normal individual and patients. From Messroghli et al. Journal of Cardiovascular Magnetic Resonance 2017;19:75. Open Access

$$ECV = \frac{\left(\frac{1}{T1\,myo_{postGd}} - \frac{1}{T1\,myo_{native}}\right)}{\left(\frac{1}{T1\,blood_{postGd}} - \frac{1}{T1\,blood_{native}}\right)} \times (100 - hematocrit)$$

Fig. 3.21 How ECV is calculated from native T1 from the myocardium and blood and after contrast injection if the haematocrit is known

in the preclinical stage of the disease. In focal and diffuse fibrosis, edema and amyloidosis, the value is increased, while it is reduced in lipid storage disorders (Anderson-Fabry disease). T1 mapping techniques allow to have a pixel by pixel map of the T1 times of the myocardium represented in a scale of colours (Fig. 3.20).

T1 mapping images are acquired in breath-hold and during the same phase of the cardiac cycle to eliminate tissue motion. Mapping techniques are either based on inversion recovery (MOLLI, ShMOLLI), saturation recovery (SASHA) or a combined approach (SAPPHIRE). Short-axis views of the LV (one slice as mid LV or three slices: basal, mid and apex) are acquired for the analysis. After injection of the contrast agent (gadolinium), T1 time is shortened, and the amount of the decrease is correlated to the amount of contrast agent that can accumulate in the extracellular space; thus it is possible to estimate the extracellular volume (ECV) by the acquisition of pre- and post-contrast T1 maps (Fig. 3.21). Post-contrast acquisition is performed at least 15 min post-contrast injection to wait for contrast equilibrium.

T2 relaxation time is especially altered by water thus in the presence of edema, and T2 mapping can be performed especially for the assessment of inflammatory diseases (myocarditis, rheumatological conditions, transplant rejection).

3.2.8 Coronary Artery Imaging

MR imaging of coronary arteries is limited by low spatial resolution and issues related to cardiac and respiratory motions.

The main clinical application of MR coronary artery imaging is the detection of abnormal origin and course of coronary arteries.

There are two main techniques:

1. Whole heart technique by a 3D volume of the heart that is acquired from the inferior border of the heart up to the bifurcation of the pulmonary artery using a respiratory navigator and the longest trigger delay (usually between 550 and 900 msec) for optimal diastolic imaging (to acquire the image at the same phase of the respiratory and cardiac cycle) is then analysed.
2. Targeted technique when the patient is able to perform a long breath-hold. A low-resolution 3D coronary survey is performed, and then the "3-point plan scan" facility is used to plan the optimal imaging plane for each coronary (typical points are placed at the ostium, mid vessel and at the distal vessel).

3.3 CMR Report

CMR reporting requires a structured approach that should include also according to guidelines of the Society of Cardiovascular Magnetic Resonance:

1. Site and equipment information
2. Patient demographics
3. Indications for the study
4. Study performance
5. Cardiovascular imaging features
6. Conclusions that summarize the CMR finding reaching a comprehensive diagnosis

Fig. 3.22 Main features that should be included in a CMR report

Cardiovascular Magnetic Resonance (CMR) Report
CMR Unit, Institution

Patients Demographics (Name, ID, Date of birth, Gender, Height, Weight)

CMR Study (Date and time, Involved personnel, Scanner details, Primary indication, List of CMR sequences, Contrast and Stress a with dosing, Vital parameters)

CMR Findings (General findings with gross vascular anatomy and connections, Specific findings on LV and RV: for each ventricle size, regional and global function and volumes with EDV, ESV, SV, EF also LV mass and all data corrected for BSA)

Summary (Main CMR finding leading to the diagnosis)

In addition any issues that affected the exam should be reported as well (e.g. arrhythmias, breath-holding problems, ECG gating issues). A sample of essential CMR report is shown in Fig. 3.22.

References

1. Sawyer-Glover A, Shellock FG. Pre-MRI procedure screening: recommendations and safety considerations for biomedical implants and devices. J Magn Resonan Imag. 2000;12(3):510.
2. Pennell DJ, Sechtem UP, Higgins CB, et al. Clinical indications for cardiovascular magnetic resonance (CMR): Consensus Panel report. Eur Heart J. 2004;25:1940–65.
3. Levine GN, Gomes AS, Arai AE, et al. Safety of magnetic resonance imaging in patients with cardiovascular devices: an American Heart Association scientific statement from the Committee on Diagnostic and Interventional Cardiac Catheterization, Council on Clinical Cardiology, and the Council on Cardiovascular Radiology and Intervention: endorsed by the American College of Cardiology Foundation, the North American Society for Cardiac Imaging, and the Society for Cardiovascular Magnetic Resonance. Circulation. 2007;116:2878–91.
4. ACCF/ACR/AHA/NASCI/SCMR. 2010 expert consensus document on cardiovascular magnetic resonance: a report of the American College of Cardiology Foundation Task Force on Expert Consensus Documents. J Am Coll Cardiol. 2010;55:2614–62.
5. Valbuena-López S, Hinojar R, Puntmann VO. Cardiovascular magnetic resonance in cardiology practice: a concise guide to image acquisition and clinical interpretation. Rev Esp Cardiol (Engl Ed). 2016;69(2):202–10.
6. Hundley WG, Bluemke D, Bogaert JG, Friedrich MG, Higgins CB, Lawson MA, McConnell MV, Raman SV, van Rossum AC, Flamm S, Kramer CM, Nagel E, Neubauer S. Society for Cardiovascular Magnetic Resonance guidelines for reporting cardiovascular magnetic resonance examinations. J Cardiovasc Magn Reson. 2009;11(1):5.

Ischemic Heart Diseases

4

Contents

4.1 CMR Imaging Techniques and Protocol for Ischemic Heart Disease

Ischemic heart diseases are the main cause of mortality in the world despite significant improvements in interventional techniques and medical therapies as well as recent reduction of ST-segment elevation myocardial infarction (STEMI) but increase of the incidence of non-ST segment elevation myocardial infarction (NSTEMI) and unstable angina [1–3]. Cardiac magnetic resonance (CMR) is able to better characterize areas of the myocardium at risk, the presence and extent of myocardial fibrosis and myocardial viability and also to detect complications either in the setting of acute or chronic ischemic heart disease. CMR is multiparametric and offers the capability of a combined study of function, kinesis and myocardial tissue characterization. For the purpose of the correct definition of ventricular segments, CMR adopts the left ventricular segmentation of the American Heart Association (Fig. 4.1).

CMR is the gold standard for the evaluation of biventricular volumes and function [1, 5]. The usual CMR sequence adopted for this evaluation is the cine sequence SSFP (steady-state free precession). STIR T2-weighted imaging allows the detection of myocardial edema that develops after 20–30 min from the onset of symptoms, and it is helpful to identify the myocardium at risk as well as evidence of

M. Imazio et al., *Learning Cardiac Magnetic Resonance*,
https://doi.org/10.1007/978-3-030-11608-8_4

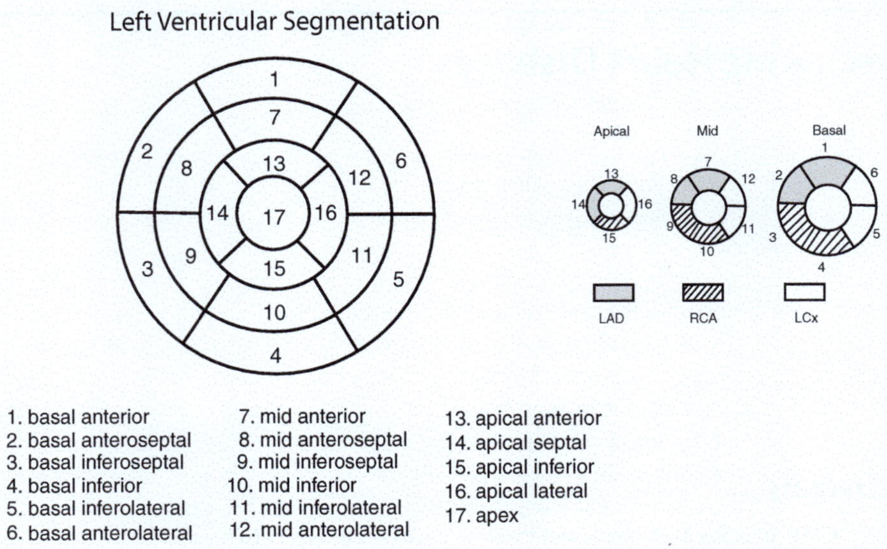

Fig. 4.1 Left ventricular segmentation according to the American Heart Association (AHA). *LAD* left anterior descending artery, *RCA* right coronary artery, *LCx* left circumflex artery

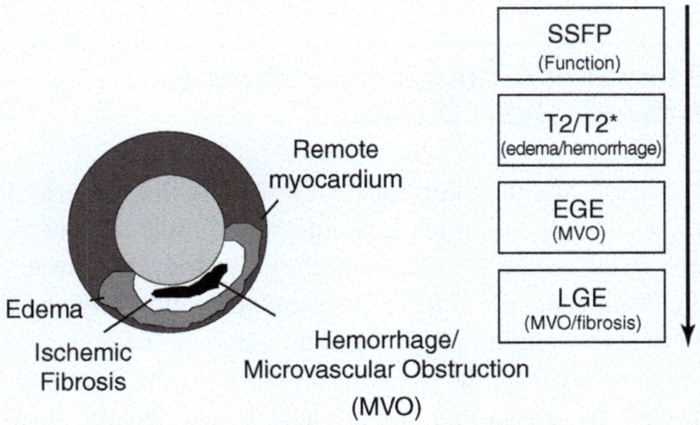

Fig. 4.2 Tissue characterization of myocardial infarction by CMR: the myocardial necrosis is depicted as scar by LGE, while the myocardium at risk is remarked as myocardial edema (T2-weighted images). Within the scar it is possible to depict hypointense areas as evidence of myocardial haemorrhage with myocardial edema or microvascular obstruction in EGE and LGE images

myocardial haemorrhage as dark ipointense areas within the myocardial edema (Fig. 4.2) [4–7].

First-passage perfusion coupled with the use of vasodilator agents (e.g. adenosine, regadenoson, dipyridamole) allows to detect stable perfusion defects when compared with basal perfusion (ischemic necrosis) and reversible defects

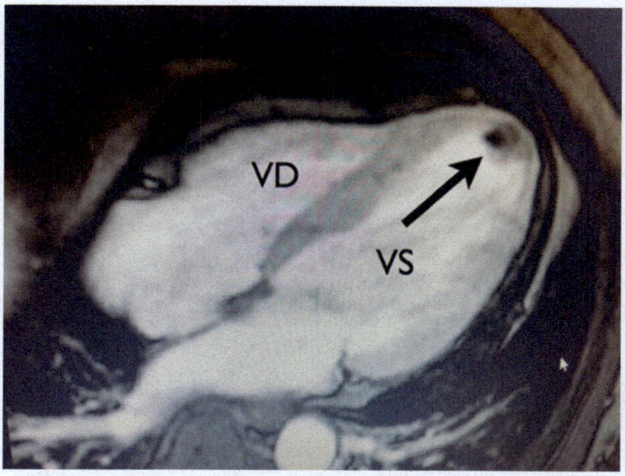

Fig. 4.3 Evidence of left ventricular thrombus at the apex of the left ventricle (LV) on EGE in the setting of anterior myocardial infarction

(inducible ischemia). Early gadolinium enhancement (EGE) allows to detect perfusion defects in the perfused myocardium as evidence of microvascular obstruction (MVO) and ventricular filling defects as evidence of ventricular thrombi (Fig. 4.3).

Late gadolinium enhancement (LGE) detects the presence of areas of extended extracellular space where gadolinium can accumulate. These areas represent myocardial edema and necrosis in the acute phase and myocardial fibrosis in the chronic phase of ischemic heart diseases. In the setting of LGE, MVO appears as areas with low signal within LGE (Figs. 4.2 and 4.4). MVO begins to be detectable few hours after an acute ischemic event and increases till 48 h reaching an equilibrium between 2 and 9 days, which represent the best time for its assessment and quantification [8]. The greater the MVO, the largest will be the scar area at 6 months [3]. Both the presence of myocardial haemorrhage and MVO predict a worse prognosis with more unfavourable remodelling at follow-up [9–11].

Ischemic LGE has a typical subendocardial or transmural distribution according to coronary artery vascularization. The extent of myocardial fibrosis can be assessed by LGE and should be considered as transmural scar extension: 1–25%, 25–50%, 51–75% and if >75%.

Myocardial viability is compromised if the extent of the scar is >50% and even more if >75%.

CMR is able to depict myocardial scar as small as those involving <1 gram of myocardial tissue. The extent of the scar is typically reduced over time due to the reabsorption of myocardial edema and hyperemia; on this basis myocardial fibrosis is evident after 3–6 months and persists after 6 months [3].

CMR allows to compare the same views with different sequences: cine SSFP (kinesis), STIR T2w images and LGE images allowing to assess the functional consequences of the myocardial scar and the extension of the myocardium at risk.

CMR allows also to detect mechanical complications of myocardial infarction (Fig. 4.5) such as septal rupture, pseudoaneurysm and aneurysm, right ventricle involvement and left ventricular thrombosis [12] and differential diagnoses with other diseases (e.g. myocarditis, MINOCA) [13–15].

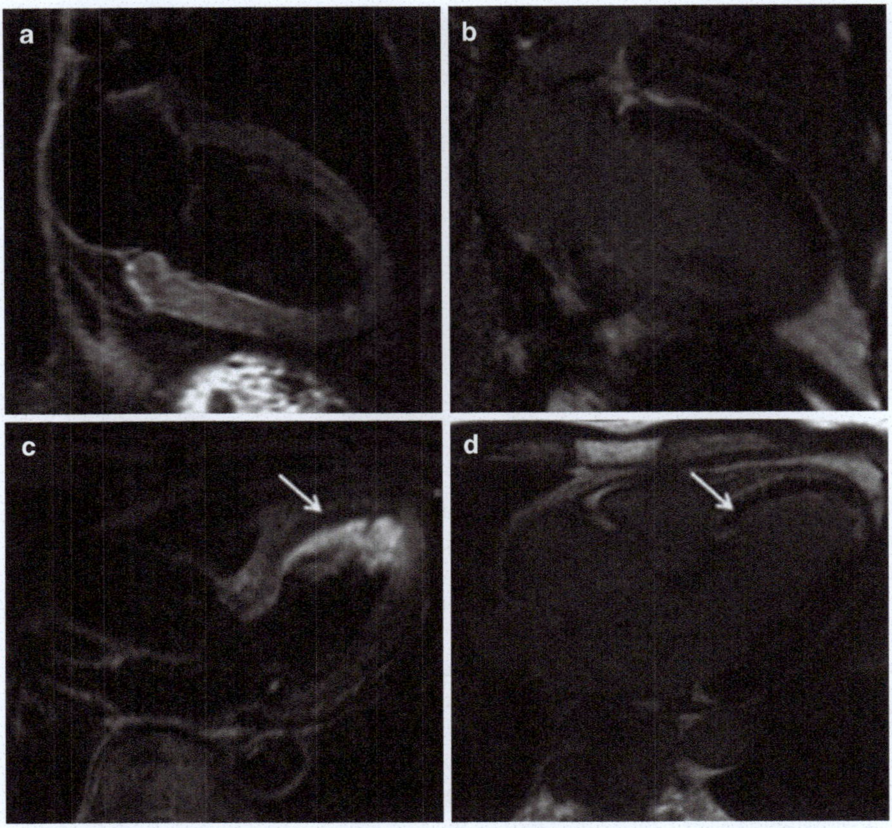

Fig. 4.4 CMR in acute coronary syndromes. Myocardial infarction: overview. T2-weighted two-chamber long-axis view showing myocardial edema in the basal to mid-cavity inferior wall (**a**) with concomitant subendocardial late gadolinium enhancement (LGE) in the post-contrast sequence (**b**) in a patient with acute subendocardial infarction in the proximal to mid right coronary artery territory. T2-weighted three-chamber long-axis view showing myocardial edema in the mid-apical anteroseptum with evidence of a hypointense core (**c**, white arrow), consistent with intramyocardial haemorrhage, in a patient with transmural infarction in the distal left anterior descending territory (**d**) with persistence of microvascular obstruction (**d**, white arrow). Four-chamber long-axis post-contrast view showing subendocardial LGE of the mid-cavity anterolateral wall (**e**). Two-chamber long-axis post-contrast view showing transmural LGE of the mid-apical inferior wall (**f**). From Baritussio A, Scatteia A, Bucciarelli-Ducci C. Role of cardiovascular magnetic resonance in acute and chronic ischemic heart disease. Int J Cardiovasc Imaging. 2018 Jan;34(1):67–80. Open access. Creative Commons Attribution 4.0 International License (http://creativecommons.org/licenses/by/4.0/)

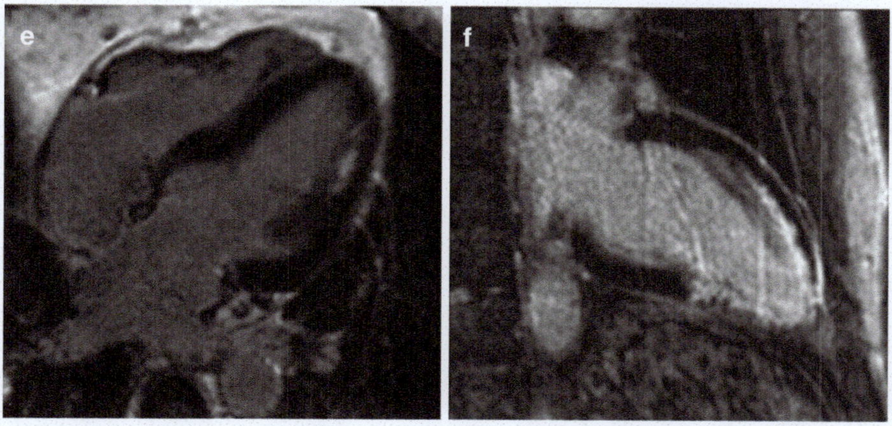

Fig. 4.4 (continued)

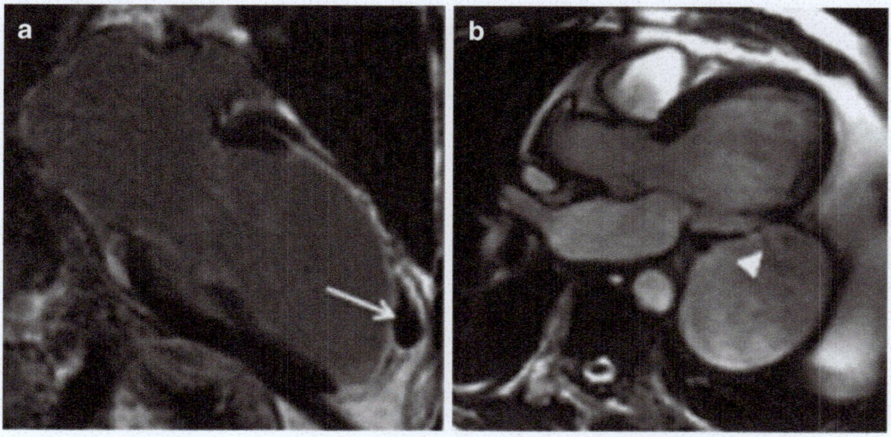

Fig. 4.5 Cases with complications of myocardial infarction: Two-chamber long-axis post-contrast sequence showing contained chronic rupture of the anterior wall (**a**, white arrow) in a patient with transmural myocardial infarction in the left anterior descending territory. Three-chamber long-axis cine sequence showing large pseudoaneurysm of the mid-cavity inferolateral wall (**b**) with evidence of flow (**b**, white arrow-head) between a "tunnel-like" connection with the left ventricle in a patient with transmural infarction in the left circumflex territory. Mid-cavity short-axis post-contrast sequence showing myocardial infarction of the papillary muscles (**c**). Mid-cavity short-axis post-contrast sequence showing myocardial infarction of the right ventricular inferior wall (**d**, black arrow) in a patient with transmural infarction in the basal inferior wall. Early (**e**) and late (**f**) four-chamber long-axis gadolinium enhancement sequences showing a large apical thrombus in a patient with transmural myocardial infarction in the distal left anterior descending territory (**f**). From Baritussio A, Scatteia A, Bucciarelli-Ducci C. Role of cardiovascular magnetic resonance in acute and chronic ischemic heart disease. Int J Cardiovasc Imaging. 2018 Jan;34(1):67–80. Open access. Creative Commons Attribution 4.0 International License (http://creativecommons.org/licenses/by/4.0/)

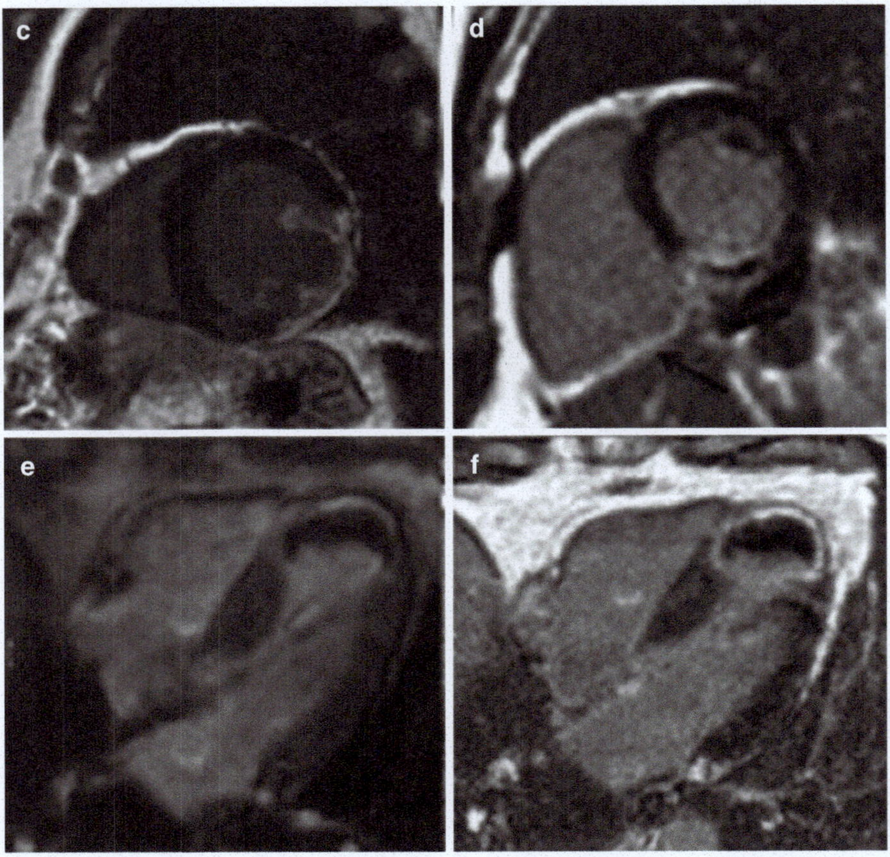

Fig. 4.5 (continued)

4.2 Comparison with Other Techniques (CMR vs. Echo vs. SPECT)

CMR and SPECT allow to identify patients who are candidate to medical therapy or subsequent coronary angiography, but CMR, due to its superior spatial resolution and capability of tissue characterization, has specific advantages over these techniques (Table 4.1):

1. Better accuracy in the evaluation of biventricular volumes and function
2. Better capability of identification and quantification of the extension of myocardial scars and viability

A patient with a negative stress CMR has a very low probability of events at follow-up making CMR a valuable and safe test and a valid alternative to SPECT.

Table 4.1 Comparison of different imaging techniques (echocardiography, cardiac magnetic resonance and SPECT) for the evaluation of ischemic heart diseases

Feature	Echocardiography	CMR	SPECT
Functional evaluation	++	+++	+
Wall thickness	++	+++	–
Evaluation of edema[a]	–	+++	–
Reperfusion[a]	–	+++	–
Myocardial viability	++	+++	+++
Thrombus	+	++	–
Inducible ischemia	+	++	++
RV evaluation	++	+++	+
Valve assessment	+++	+	–

RV Right ventricle
[a]Evaluation of myocardial edema and microvascular obstruction (MVO)

Table 4.2 Mean values of sensitivity and specificity for different tests in the evaluation of inducible myocardial ischemia in chronic ischemic heart diseases

	Sensitivity (%)	Specificity (%)
Exercise testing	60–65	70
Stress echocardiography	75–80	75–90
SPECT	67–88	73–85
Stress CMR	85–90	75–85
Coronary CT	80–85	70–75

The evaluation of myocardial viability and the extension of myocardial scar and the presence of possible signs of late reperfusion (myocardial haemorrhage and MVO) allow to identify patients with an unfavourable remodelling and worse prognosis. A greater extent of LGE (usually identified with an intensity > +5 SD compared with remote myocardium) and especially perilesional fibrosis (LGE intensity between 2 and 3 times SD compared with remote myocardium) may allow to identify a higher arrhythmic risk [3].

Stress CMR is now a well-established alternative method for the evaluation of patients with chronic ischemic heart diseases [16]. In the prospective study, CE-MARC stress CMR has been compared with SPECT [17]. Stress CMR has shown a higher sensibility (87 vs. 67%), similar specificity (83%) but higher diagnostic accuracy (89 vs. 74%) compared with SPECT [17]. The study MR-IMPACT II [18] has also confirmed the higher diagnostic accuracy of CMR compared with SPECT (respectively, 75 vs. 60%). In a systematic review, the overall sensitivity of CMR was 89%; specificity was 76% if the gold standard for the evaluation of patients has been coronary angiography [19]. Such values improve if the gold standard is the fractional flow reserve (FFR) with overall sensitivity up to 90% and specificity up to 87% [20]. A summary of current available data on sensitivity and specificity of different techniques is reported in Table 4.2.

On this basis, stress CMR is now included for the evaluation of patients with suspicion of chronic ischemic heart disease in international guidelines [21–23].

In 2013 ESC guidelines [21], stress CMR is included in the first options for the assessment of patients with suspected angina and intermediate probability of disease (15–85%) as well as exercise testing, stress echocardiography, SPECT and coronary CT (Table 4.3).

Table 4.3 Indication to stress CMR according to 2013 ESC guidelines [21]

2013 ESC guidelines
1. Stress CMR is indicated as initial test for the diagnosis of ischemic heart disease in patients with an intermediate[a] probability of disease (Class I)
2. Stress CMR can be used for prognostic stratification with clinical evaluation (Class I)
3. Stress CMR is indicated in patients with known CAD and new or recurrent symptoms if the determination of the localization and extent of ischemia can affect the subsequent clinical decision to treat (Class I)

[a]15–85%

On the contrary, American guidelines prefer exercise testing and SPECT, and stress CMR is a second option due to consideration on the availability and more physiologic type of stress testing [22]. In the more recent study CE-MARC [24], a strategy based on the evaluation of patients with stress CMR or SPECT reduced the need for unnecessary coronary angiography (=coronary angiography with absence of significant coronary artery disease) compared with coronary CT, as indicated as first choice in the NICE guidelines [23]. However no significant advantages were detected in the use of a specific strategy between stress CMR and SPECT.

4.3 Case: Assessment of Myocardial Viability and Complications

A 50-year-old man, smoker, with no previous history of cardiovascular diseases is referred for CMR as a late presentation for anterior STEMI.

On CMR, cine imaging showed a non-dilated LV with wall motion abnormalities with apical, mid-apical septal, anterior and anterolateral akinesia and mild reduction of systolic function (EF 45%). After contrast injection, EGE showed a ventricular apical thrombus (see black arrow on Fig. 4.6) and evidence of subendocardial LGE with variable extension >50% of wall thickness and apical transmurality (Fig. 4.6).

This case shows that CMR is able to provide combined information on function, complications and localization and extension of scar useful for viability considerations.

4.4 Key Points and Protocols

- CMR has a better spatial resolution and capability of tissue characterization compared with other imaging techniques in the evaluation of ischemic heart disease.
- CMR is the gold standard for the evaluation of biventricular volumes and function and allows a better and more accurate study of wall motion abnormalities, localization and extent of myocardial scars as well as evaluation of the myocardium at risk (assessed by myocardial edema), late reperfusion (assessed by myocardial haemorrhage and MVO) and complications (thrombi, mechanical complications, RV involvement).

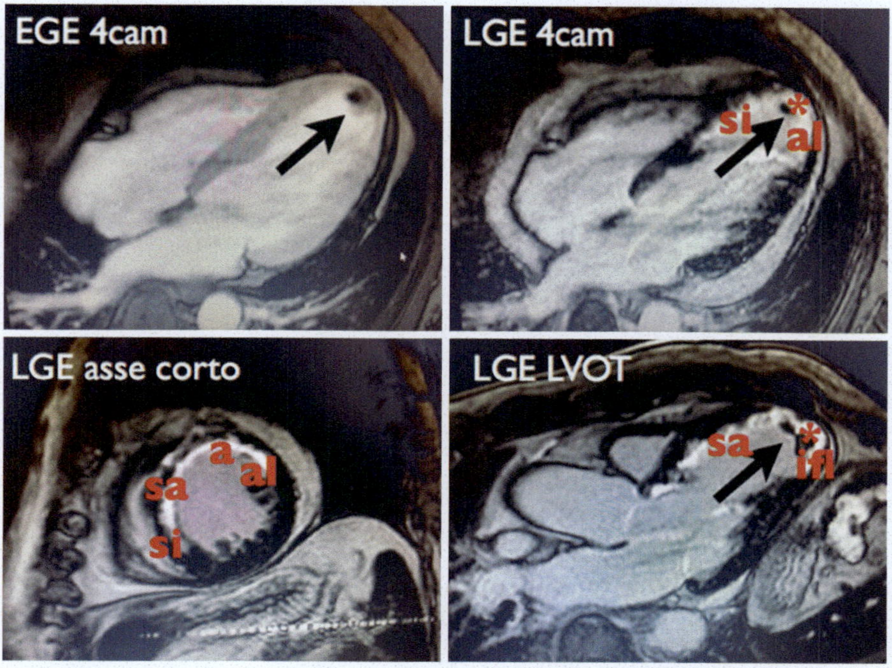

Fig. 4.6 A case of anterior STEMI with late presentation and evidence of LV apical thrombus on EGE 4cam and LGE 4cam (see black arrow) and subendocardial LGE with variable extension >50% in apical, mid-apical septal, anterior and anterolateral segments

- CMR T2-weighted imaging allows the detection of myocardial edema that identifies the myocardium at risk in the setting of acute ischemic heart disease.
- LGE allows to localize and quantify the extension of myocardial scar.
- Stress CMR is a first-choice alternative for the evaluation of patients with suspected CAD and intermediate probability of disease as well as patients with known CAD and new symptoms.
- A complete protocol for the evaluation of a patient with ischemic heart disease includes cine sequences, STIR T2w imaging, stress perfusion (according to the clinical indication) and early and late gadolinium enhancement (see also Table 4.4).

Table 4.4 Standard protocol for the evaluation of a patient with ischemic heart disease

Sequence	Data
Cine SSFP	Evaluation of biventricular volumes and function (segmental and global)
STIR T2-weighted	Evaluation of myocardial edema (myocardium at risk), myocardial haemorrhage within edema (hypodense signals within edema for reduction of T2 by iron within haemoglobin)
Perfusion	Basale and stress CMR (according to clinical indication)
EGE	Evaluation of ventricular thrombi and microvascular obstruction (MVO) as hypodense signals within the scar
LGE	Evaluation of the scar: subendocardial with variable extension up to transmurality, possible evaluation of MVO within the scar

EGE Early gadolinium enhancement, *LGE* late gadolinium enhancement

References

1. Dastidar AG, Rodrigues JC, Baritussio A, Bucciarelli-Ducci C. MRI in the assessment of ischaemic heart disease. Heart. 2016;102(3):239–52.
2. McAlindon E, Pufulete M, Lawton C, Angelini GD, Bucciarelli-Ducci C. Quantification of infarct size and myocardium at risk: evaluation of different techniques and its implications. Eur Heart J Cardiovasc Imaging. 2015;16(7):738–46.
3. Baritussio A, Scatteia A, Bucciarelli-Ducci C. Role of cardiovascular magnetic resonance in acute and chronic ischemic heart disease. Int J Cardiovasc Imaging. 2018;34(1):67–80.
4. Aquaro GD, Di Bella G, Castelletti S, et al. Clinical recommendation of cardiac magnetic resonance, part I: ischemic and valvular heart disease: a position paper of the working group "Applicazioni della Risonanza Magnetica" of the Italian Society of Cardiology. J Cardiovasc Med. 2017;18:197–208.
5. Hoffmann R, von Bardeleben S, Kasprzak JD, et al. Analysis of regional left ventricular function by cineventriculography, cardiac magnetic resonance imaging, and unenhanced and contrast-enhanced echocardiography: a multicenter comparison of methods. J Am Coll Cardiol. 2006;47:121–8.
6. Aletras AH, Tilak GS, Natanzon A, et al. Retrospective determination of the area at risk for reperfused acute myocardial infarction with T2-weighted cardiac magnetic resonance imaging: histopathological and displacement encoding with stimulated echoes (DENSE) functional validations. Circulation. 2006;113(15):1865–70.
7. Eitel I, Friedrich MG. T2-weighted cardiovascular magnetic resonance in acute cardiac disease. J Cardiovasc Magn Reson. 2011;13(1):13.
8. Beek AM, van Rossum AC. Cardiovascular magnetic resonance imaging in patients with acute myocardial infarction. Heart. 2010;96:237–43.
9. Husser O, Monmeneu JV, Sanchis J, et al. Cardiovascular magnetic resonance-derived intramyocardial hemorrhage after STEMI: influence on long-term prognosis, adverse left ventricular remodeling and relationship with microvascular obstruction. Int J Cardiol. 2013;167(5):2047–54.
10. Romero J, Lupercio F, Carlos J, et al. Microvascular obstruction detected by cardiac MRI after AMI for the prediction of LV remodeling and MACE: a meta-analysis of prospective trials. Int J Cardiol. 2016;202:344–8.
11. Kidambi A, Mather AN, Motwani M, Swoboda P, Uddin A, Greenwood JP, Plein S. The effect of microvascular obstruction and intramyocardial hemorrhage on contractile recovery in reperfused myocardial infarction: insights from cardiovascular magnetic resonance. J Cardiovasc Magn Reson. 2013;15:58.
12. Flavian A, Carta F, Thuny F, et al. Cardiac MRI in the diagnosis of complications of myocardial infarction. Diagn Interv Imaging. 2012;93(7–8):578–85.
13. Dastidar AG, Rodrigues JCL, Ahmed N, Baritussio A, Bucciarelli-Ducci C. The role of cardiac MRI in patients with troponin-positive chest pain and unobstructed coronary arteries. Curr Cardiovasc Imaging Rep. 2015;8(8):28.
14. Tornvall P, Gerbaud E, Behaghel A, et al. Myocarditis or "true" infarction by cardiac magnetic resonance in patients with a clinical diagnosis of myocardial infarction without obstructive coronary disease: a meta-analysis of individual patient data. Atherosclerosis. 2015;241(1):87–91.
15. Mahrholdt H, Wagner A, Judd RM, Sechtem U, Kim RJ. Delayed enhancement cardiovascular magnetic resonance assessment of non-ischaemic cardiomyopathies. Eur Heart J. 2005;26(15):1461–74.
16. Motwani M, Swoboda PP, Plein S, Greenwood JP. Role of cardiovascular magnetic resonance in the management of patients with stable coronary artery disease. Heart. 2018;104(11):888–94. https://doi.org/10.1136/heartjnl-2017-311658.
17. Greenwood JP, Maredia N, Younger JF, et al. Cardiovascular magnetic resonance and single-photon emission computed tomography for diagnosis of coronary heart disease (CE-MARC): a prospective trial. Lancet. 2012;379:453–60.

18. Schwitter J, Wacker CM, Wilke N, et al. Superior diagnostic performance of perfusion cardiovascular magnetic resonance versus SPECT to detect coronary artery disease: the secondary endpoints of the multicenter multivendor MR-IMPACT II (Magnetic Resonance Imaging for Myocardial Perfusion Assessment in Coronary Artery Disease Trial). J Cardiovasc Magn Reson. 2012;14:61.
19. Jaarsma C, Leiner T, Bekkers SC, et al. Diagnostic performance of noninvasive myocardial perfusion imaging using single-photon emission computed tomography, cardiac magnetic resonance, and positron emission tomography imaging for the detection of obstructive coronary artery disease: a meta-analysis. J Am Coll Cardiol. 2012;59:1719–28.
20. Li M, Zhou T, Yang LF, et al. Diagnostic accuracy of myocardial magnetic resonance perfusion to diagnose ischemic stenosis with fractional flow reserve as reference: systematic review and meta-analysis. JACC Cardiovasc Imaging. 2014;7:1098–105.
21. Montalescot G, Sechtem U, Achenbach S, et al. 2013 ESC guidelines on the management of stable coronary artery disease: the task force on the management of stable coronary artery disease of the European Society of Cardiology. Eur Heart J. 2013;34:2949–3003.
22. Fihn SD, Gardin JM, Abrams J, et al. 2012 ACCF/AHA/ACP/AATS/PCNA/SCAI/STS guideline for the diagnosis and management of patients with stable ischemic heart disease: a report of the American College of Cardiology Foundation/American Heart Association task force on practice guidelines, and the American College of Physicians, American Association for Thoracic Surgery, Preventive Cardiovascular Nurses Association, Society for Cardiovascular Angiography and Interventions, and Society of Thoracic Surgeons. Circulation. 2012;126:e354–471.
23. National Institute for Health and Care Excellence (NICE). CG95 Chest pain of recent onset 2016. http://guidance.nice.org.uk/CG95. Accessed Sep 2017.
24. Greenwood JP, Ripley DP, Berry C, et al. Effect of care guided by cardiovascular magnetic resonance, myocardial perfusion scintigraphy, or nice guidelines on subsequent unnecessary angiography rates: the CE-MARC 2 randomized clinical trial. JAMA. 2016;316:1051–60.

Cardiomyopathies

5

Contents

5.1 Introduction and CMR Advantages in the Study of Cardiomyopathies

Cardiac magnetic resonance (CMR) is the gold standard for the evaluation of biventricular volumes and function as well as non-invasive tissue characterization of myocardial edema and fibrosis; on this basis, CMR is an important second-level imaging technique for the study of cardiomyopathies (CMPs) that are a common indication for this type of diagnostic test [1]. In the EuroCMR registry, about one-third of CMR tests were performed to evaluate patients with suspected or known myocarditis and CMPs [2, 3].

M. Imazio et al., *Learning Cardiac Magnetic Resonance*,
https://doi.org/10.1007/978-3-030-11608-8_5

In the present chapter, we will discuss and review CMR criteria and findings in the study of CMPs following a simple classification:

1. Dilated cardiomyopathies (DCM)
2. Genetic cardiomyopathies (hypertrophic CMP, LV non-compaction cardiomyopathy, Becker and Duchenne muscular dystrophy, RV arrhythmogenic CMP)
3. Inflammatory cardiomyopathies (sarcoidosis, CMPs associated with systemic inflammatory syndromes)
4. Infiltrative CMPs (amyloidosis, iron overload CMP, Anderson-Fabry disease)

Takotsubo syndrome will be discussed at the end since it is usually erroneously included in cardiomyopathies.

5.2 Dilated Cardiomyopathy (DCM)

DCM is the final manifestation of several forms of non-ischemic damage. In the setting of DCM, CMR allows:

1. A more precise anatomical (T1w imaging) and functional evaluation (cine sequences)
2. To rule out myocarditis as precipitating cause of ventricular dysfunction by STIR T2w imaging and EGE and LGE (in the acute setting of myocarditis, ventricles are not dilated and may have increased thickness because of myocardial oedema)
3. To rule out an ischemic cause of LV dysfunction (previous or new myocardial infarctions) by LGE (ischemic pattern of scar is subendocardial or transmural)
4. To better study the right ventricle (RV)
5. To assess the presence and extent of either ischemic or non-ischemic scars (e.g. septal midwall in true DCM) that may identify patients at high risk of death, arrhythmias and worsening LV function

Case 1. DCM with septal midwall scar (Fig. 5.1). A 60-year-old man with a known DCM is studied by CMR. On LGE imaging a non-ischemic midwall septal scar was identified.

In DCM, CMR testing may only show LV dilatation and dysfunction without signs of infiltration, myocardial edema and scar. A common pattern identified in 25 to 30% of cases is a non-ischemic septal midwall scar that identifies a subgroup of patients with a worse prognosis with an increased risk of arrhythmias, death and especially sudden cardiac death independently from the degree of LV dysfunction [1, 4, 5].

Increased interstitial fibrosis without scars can be also evaluated by CMR [6]. T1-mapping techniques allow to identify patients with increased interstitial fibrosis by simply the evaluation of T1 (without use of contrast agents) or by estimation of the extracellular space volume (ECV) by the use of gadolinium contrast agents (Figs. 5.2 and 5.3).

A subgroup of DCM is associated with Becker and, especially, Duchenne muscular dystrophy. Less than 10% of these patients may have a reduced ejection

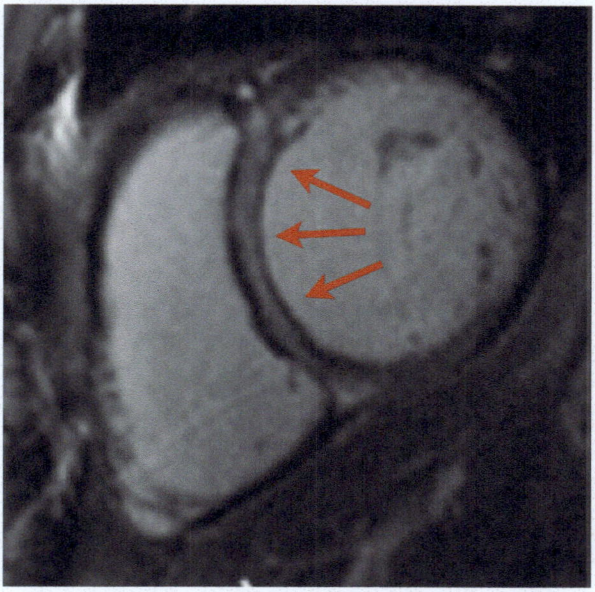

Fig. 5.1 A patient with DCM and severe LV dysfunction with evidence of non-ischemic midwall fibrosis at the level of IV septum (see red arrows)

fraction (EF) below 35%. CMR may be helpful to identify early forms with cardiovascular involvement before reduction of the EF by the use of strain. More than 1/3 of patients with Duchenne muscular dystrophy have non-ischemic LGE with a typical localization in the lateral subepicardium. Such type of LGE is associated with an increased risk of progression towards LV dysfunction and death [1].

5.3 Genetic Cardiomyopathies

Genetic CMPs included CMPs due to genetic mutations. The most common form is hypertrophic CMP (HCM).

5.3.1 Hypertrophic Cardiomyopathy (HCM)

HCM is a genetic CMP caused by genetic mutations affecting sarcomeric proteins with a prevalent autosomal dominant transmission (but also other modalities of transmission have been demonstrated, although less common: X-linked and recessive). It is now one of the most common genetic diseases with a prevalence now revised to >1/500 and up to 1/200–1/300 [7]. The disease is usually evident from the adolescence with an overall risk of death <1% but higher in series from referral centres (3–6%). According to 2014 ESC guidelines [8], CMR should be considered in the initial evaluation of patients with HCM since this diagnostic technique is superior to echocardiography in the evaluation of specific forms of hypertrophy (apical, anterolateral), complications such as aneurysms, thrombi and markers of the diseases (e.g. abnormalities of papillary muscles, crypts) [9–14]. CMR is also able to demonstrate non-ischemic scars in >1/3 of patients by LGE, typically the midwall in

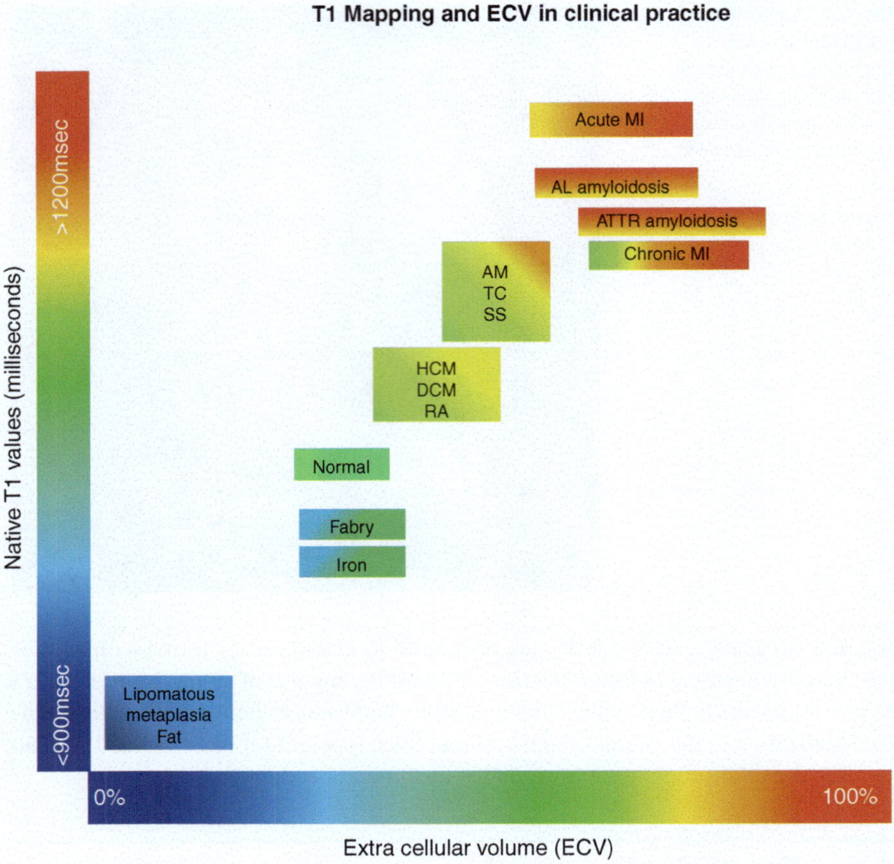

Fig. 5.2 Interstitial fibrosis is responsible of increased values of T1 and ECV. These techniques are now emerging but still not fully integrated in common clinical routine since to be well standardized. From Messroghli et al. Journal of Cardiovascular Magnetic Resonance (2017) 19:75(6). Open Access

$$ECV = \frac{\left(\frac{1}{T1myo_{postGd}} - \frac{1}{T1myo_{native}}\right)}{\left(\frac{1}{T1blood_{postGd}} - \frac{1}{T1blood_{native}}\right)} \times (100 - hematocrit)$$

Fig. 5.3 Formula for the estimation of ECV from values of myocardial T1 (T1myo) and blood T1 (T1blood) before and after contrast injection if the value of blood haematocrit is known. The principle is that contrast agent may occupy a greater extent of extracellular space if interstitial fibrosis is present, thus affecting T1. Native T1 is increased with fibrosis

hypertrophied areas, at the level of RV insertions on the interventricular septum. CMR is able to accurately measure wall thickness and myocardial mass and help in the differential diagnosis (e.g. infiltrative CMPs such as amyloidosis, Anderson-Fabry disease) [9–13].

The indications to CMR in HCM are summarized in Table 5.1.

Table 5.1 HCM: indications for CMR according to 2014 ESC guidelines [8]

Indication	Class	LOE
It is recommended that CMR studies be performed and interpreted by teams experienced in cardiac imaging and in the evaluation of heart muscle disease	I	C
In the absence of contraindications, CMR with LGE is recommended in patients with suspected HCM who have inadequate echocardiographic windows, in order to confirm the diagnosis	I	B
In the absence of contraindications, CMR with LGE should be considered in patients fulfilling diagnostic criteria for HCM, to assess cardiac anatomy, ventricular function and the presence and extent of myocardial fibrosis	IIa	B
CMR with LGE imaging should be considered in patients with suspected apical hypertrophy or aneurysm	IIa	C
CMR with LGE imaging should be considered in patients with suspected cardiac amyloidosis	IIa	C
CMR with LGE may be considered before septal alcohol ablation or myectomy, to assess the extent and distribution of hypertrophy and myocardial fibrosis	IIb	C

LOE level of evidence, *Class I* indicated, *II* most opinions agree (IIa) or generally agree for (IIb), *III* contraindicated

A CMR protocol for the evaluation of HCM should include cine sequences (evaluation of the entity and distribution of the hypertrophy, biventricular study of volumes, function and masses), and a specific care should be devoted to assess LV outflow tract (LVOT), if a dynamic gradient is present as well as systolic anterior motion (SAM) of anterior leaflet of the mitral valve (phase contrast imaging may be helpful to depict the presence of a dynamic gradient in the LVOT) and non-ischemic myocardial scars on LGE. The CMR report should include detailed informations regarding:

1. Volumes, masses and biventricular function
2. Wall thickness and segmental LV function
3. Presence or absence of dynamic obstruction in the LVOT and SAM
4. Presence and extension of myocardial scars

In these patients, risk factors for sudden cardiac death (SCD) are clinical (positive family history, syncope, nonsustained VT, hypotension on exertion) but also linked to imaging:

1. Massive hypertrophy >30 mm (telediastolic thickness)
2. Presence and extension of LGE [15]
3. Presence of dynamic obstruction in LVOT

CMR findings for HCM include:

1. Localized LV hypertrophy (>15 mm or septal/later thickness ratio > 1.3). CMR is better than echocardiography to identify apical and lateral forms of hypertrophy.
2. Hypokinesis of hypertrophied segments.
3. Presence of crypts, a marker of disease that can also be found in carriers of mutations, who may have not developed asymmetric hypertrophy yet.
4. Presence of non-ischemic scars (LGE) in hypertrophied segments.

Cases with different forms of LV hypertrophy (septal, midwall, apical and symmetrical) are illustrated in Fig. 5.4. Crypts are discrete fissurations of compacted myocardium involving >50% of the wall thickness. They are not uncommon in an unselected population (about 6% of patients), but are more common in patients with HCM (up to 12% of patients), and especially in carriers of HCM mutations (up to 24%). The most common localization of crypts is the inferior wall and especially the basal portion of this wall that accounts for >2/3 of reported cases (Fig. 5.5) [14].

Non-ischemic scars are usually intramyocardial in HCM affecting segments with pathological hypertrophy. A non-specific pattern can be also observed at the junctional points of the right ventricle (RV) on the interventricular septum (IVS) (Fig. 5.6). In a recent systematic review of the prognostic meaning of LGE involving almost 3000 patients with HCM, the presence of LGE was associated with 3.4 times increased risk of SCD, increased risk of overall mortality and cardiovascular mortality and increased risk of heart failure [15].

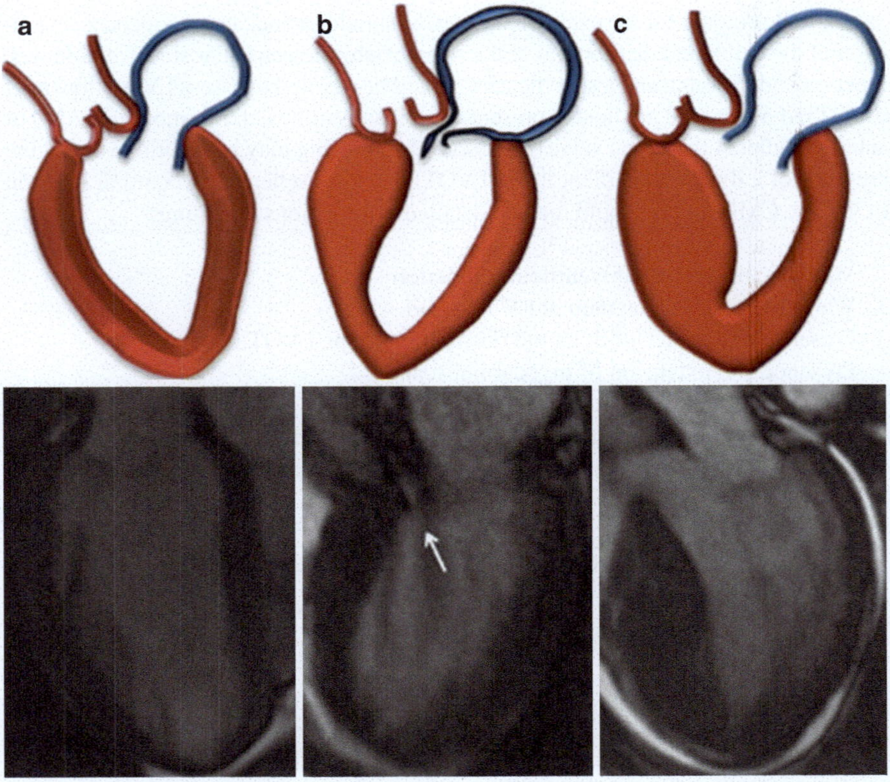

Fig. 5.4 Cases with different forms of LV hypertrophy in HCM: (**A**) normal myocardium, (**B**) septal hypertrophy with SAM, (**C**) septal hypertrophy, (**D**) mid-ventricular hypertrophy, (**E**) apical hypertrophy and (**F**) symmetric hypertrophy. From Noureldin et al. Journal of Cardiovascular Magnetic Resonance 2012, 14:17. Open access

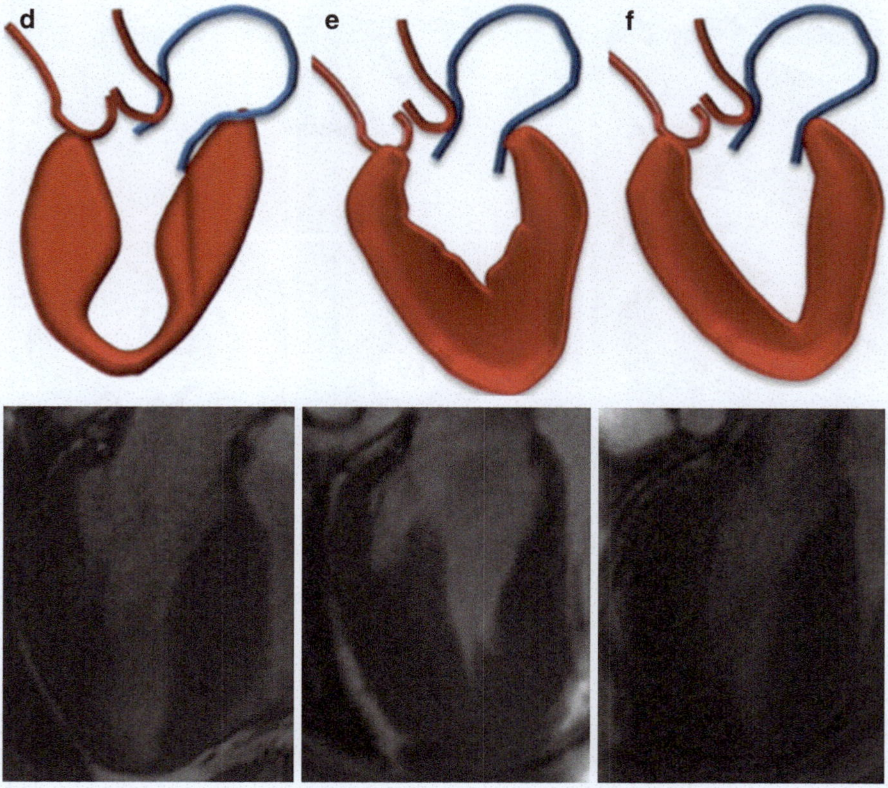

Fig. 5.4 (continued)

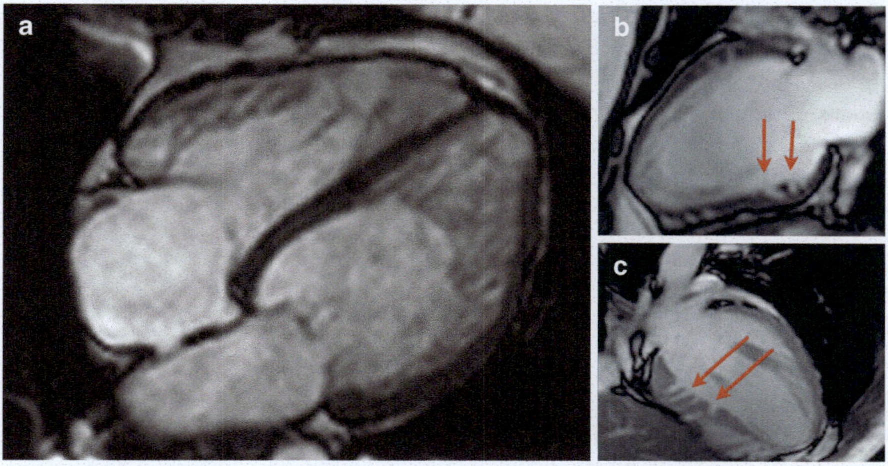

Fig. 5.5 Cases with LV non-compaction (panel **a**) and two different cases with myocardial crypts involving the basal segment of the inferior wall (panels **b** and **c**). Tratto da Child et al. Journal of Cardiovascular Magnetic Resonance 2014, 16:66. Open access

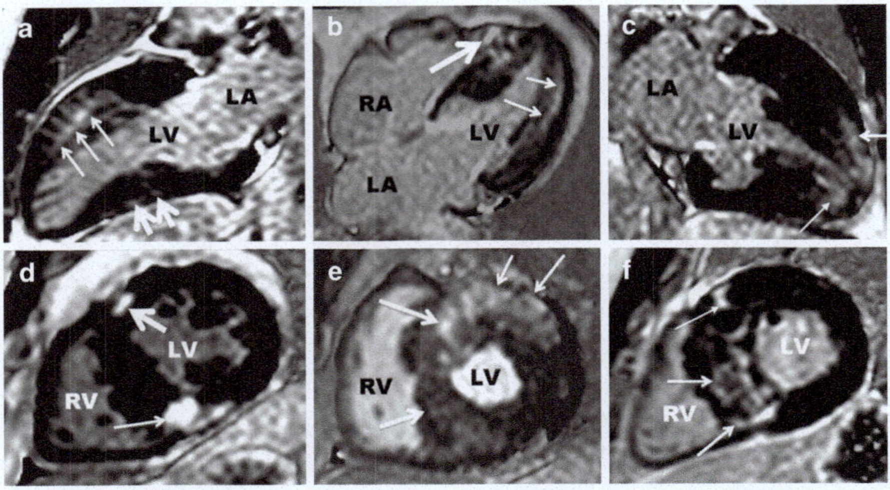

Fig. 5.6 Different patterns of hypertrophy in HCM: (**a**) anterior intramyocardial and inferior subepicardial LGE, (**b**) midwall LGE with extension towards the RV, (**c**) apical LGE, (**d**) LGE at the insertion points of the RV on the IVS, (**e**) massive LGE with almost transmural appearance and (**f**) septal LGE at the insertion of the RV on the IVS. From Maron Journal of Cardiovascular Magnetic Resonance 2012, 14:13. Open access

5.3.1.1 Case with HCM

A 42-year-old woman, asymptomatic, with normal blood pressure, presented to echo lab for a check-up. She had family history of cardiac sudden death. The echo revealed concentric left ventricular hypertrophy (IVS thickness 22 mm, inferior wall thickness 21 mm), normal ejection fraction and no valvular diseases. The patient was recommended to perform cardiac MR in order to evaluate myocardial tissue.

The MR images on SSFP sequences confirmed normal LVEF and IVS thickening of 24 mm and inferior wall thickening of 22 mm (Fig. 5.7, panels a and b). LGE images demonstrated a non-ischemic LGE in inferior midwall (see white arrows and panels c and d). In conclusion, cardiac MR diagnosed HCM with fibrosis. LGE identifies patients at elevated risk. In this case ECG Holter monitoring was performed and did not show any arrhythmias. Beta blockers were recommended, and it was decided to have a short-term clinical follow-up.

5.3.2 Left Ventricular Non-compaction (LVNC)

Left ventricular non-compaction (LVNC) is a CMP attributed to incomplete or aberrant development of normal myocardium. A genetic component can be detected in about 1/3 of cases with mutations involving sarcomeric or cytoskeletal proteins [1, 16]. The current European classification of CMP includes LVNC in unclassified forms [17].

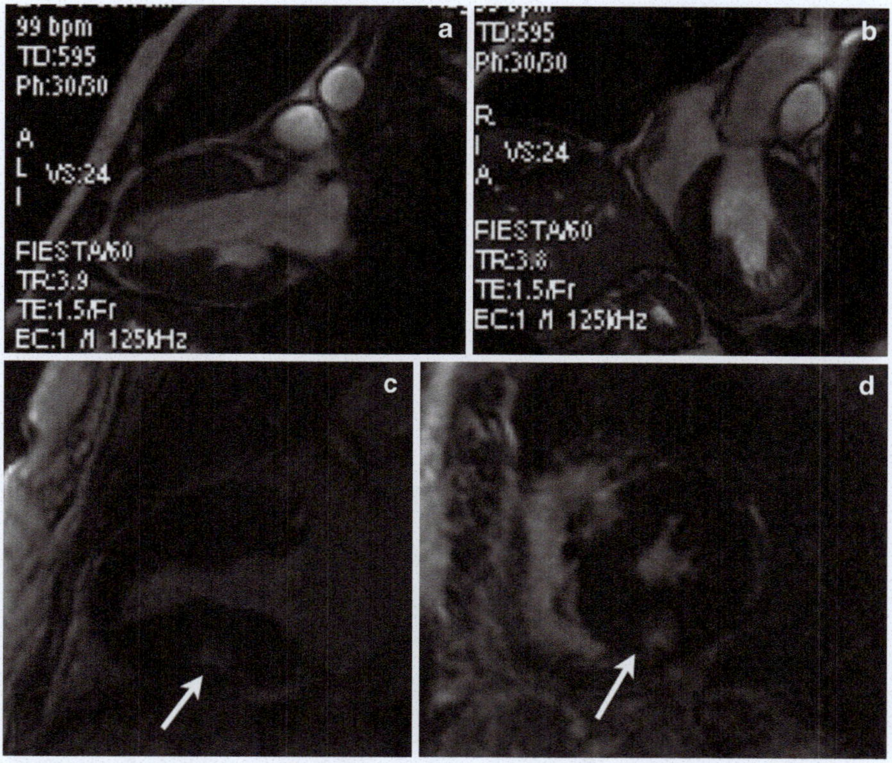

Fig. 5.7 A case with symmetric HCM (panels **a**, **b**) and non-ischemic LGE in the inferior wall (panels **c**, **d**)

On autopsy, LVNC is diagnosed by comparison of non-compacted (NC) vs. compacted (C) areas of the myocardium: the diagnosis is reached if NC/C > 2.

Possible complications of LVNC are represented by ventricular thrombi, ventricular dysfunction, heart failure and arrhythmias. LVNC usually affects apical and lateral portions of the LV. In a recent study evaluating the clinical evolution of LVNC determined by CMR in apparently normal subjects, there were no complications and evolution during a 10-year follow-up [18].

CMR has an excellent contrast well depicting LV cavity and endocardial borders and thus allows the diagnosis of LVNC. Different diagnostic criteria have been proposed using echocardiography or CMR (see Table 5.2) [19–22]. The simplest criterion is the measure of the telediastolic ratio of NC/C in long-axis scans of the LV according to Petersen criterion: LVNC is diagnosed if NC/C > 2.3 (Fig. 5.8). Jacquier criterion is based on the assessment of masses: LVNC is diagnosed if NC mass is >20% [21]. More recently, Stacey et al. have proposed to evaluate the telesystolic ratio of NC/C in short axis: the diagnosis is reached if NC/C > 2 [22].

An example of estimation of LVNC by Petersen criteria is illustrated in the case of Fig. 5.8.

Table 5.2 Different diagnostic criteria for LVNC [19–22]

	Jenni [19]	Petersen [20]	Jacquier [21]	Stacey [22]
Diagnostic test	Echocardiography	CMR	CMR	CMR
Scan	Parasternal SA	3 Long axis scans cine SSFP	Short axis scan cine SSFP	Short axis scan cine SSFP
Cardiac phase	Telesystole	Telediastole	Telediastole	Telesystole
Criterion	NC/C > 2	NC/C > 2.3	NC mass > 20%	NC/C > 2
Sensitivity	n.a.	86%	94%	n.a.
Specificity	n.a.	99%	94%	n.a.

SA short axis, *n.a.* not available

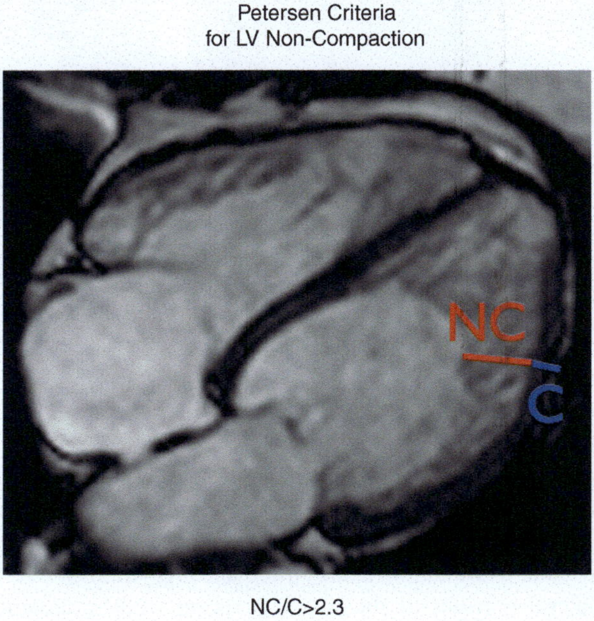

Fig. 5.8 An illustrative case of LVNC evaluated by Petersen criteria: the telediastolic ratio of NC/C is calculated in a long-axis scan of the LV (in this case four-chamber scan of the ventricles). A diagnosis of LVNC is made in this case since the ratio is >2.3

The detection of LVNC is often a reason of concern. In athletes, LVNC is reported in 1–4% of cases, but it is pathological only in 0.1% of cases because of concomitant LV dysfunction (EF < 50%) or positive family history [23]. LVNC is not associated with a worse prognosis in asymptomatic patients with preserved LV function [18]. If LV dysfunction is present, patients should be treated according to heart failure guidelines; on the contrary, if asymptomatic and without a positive family history (CMP, SCD, muscular dystrophy), the patient should be reassured, and follow-up is even not recommended (Fig. 5.9).

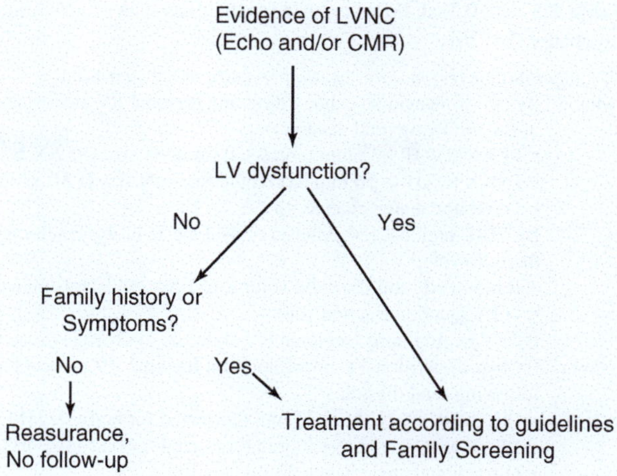

Fig. 5.9 Suggested management for patients with a new diagnosis of LVNC. Family history includes CMPs, SCD, muscular dystrophies and congenital heart diseases. Symptoms are related to thrombi, LV dysfunction of heart failure, syncope and arrhythmias

5.3.3 Right Ventricle Arrhythmogenic Cardiomyopathy

RV arrhythmogenic CMP is a genetic CMP, mainly with an autosomal dominant transmission that is responsible for RV involvement with dilatation and/or global or segmental dysfunction in most cases. Such RV involvement can be documented by CMR.

Current CMR criteria for the diagnosis of this CMP only include the evaluation of the segmental and global RV function (see Table 5.3) and have a higher sensitivity and specificity compared with older ones [24, 25].

RV arrhythmogenic CMP is a progressive disease associated with an elevated risk of major ventricular arrhythmias that can be life-threatening. In 50–60% of cases, a mutation involving can be identified: mutations involve desmosome proteins responsible for myocyte adhesion. The diagnosis is reached combining clinical, genetic and imaging criteria. The left ventricle can be involved in >50% of cases; on this basis, the term "arrhythmogenic CMP" has been proposed to include the possible biventricular involvement [26].

ECG is altered in the early phases of the diseases with negative T waves on right precordial leads (V1–V2); arrhythmias originating from the RV have a typical morphology with LBB and superior axis.

CMR is helpful to assess segmental and global function of the RV with telediastolic volume. According to diagnostic criteria, CMR alone is not sufficient for the diagnosis, and the integration with other criteria is necessary to reach the diagnosis [26]. Fibro-fatty or fibrous replacement of the myocardium can be assessed by CMR; it is not included in current diagnostic criteria and may involve the LV.

A case-example of arrhythmogenic right ventricular cardiomyopathy is reported (ARVC; Fig. 5.10). A 67-year-old man had evidence of negative T waves on V1 to V4

Table 5.3 2010 Task Force criteria for the diagnosis of arrhythmogenic right ventricular cardiomyopathy [24, 26]

I. Global and/or regional dysfunction and structural alterations	
Major	By two-dimensional echocardiogram, regional RV akinesia, dyskinesia or aneurysm and one of the following (end diastole): • PLAX RVOT ≥32 mm (corrected for body size [PLAX/BSA] ≥ 19 mm/m^2) • PSAX RVOT ≥ 36 mm (corrected for body size [PSAX/BSA] ≥ 21 mm/m^2) • O fractional area change ≤33% By MRI: regional RV akinesia or dyskinesia or dyssynchronous RV contraction and one of the following: • Ratio of RV end-diastolic volume to BSA ≥ 110 mL/m^2 (male) or ≥100 mL/m^2 (female) • O RV ejection fraction ≤40% By RV angiography: regional RV akinesia, dyskinesia or aneurysm
Minor	By two-dimensional echocardiogram: regional RV akinesia or dyskinesia and one of the following (end diastole): • PLAX RVOT ≥29 to <32 mm (corrected for body size [PLAX/BSA] ≥ 16 to <19 mm/m^2) • PSAX RVOT ≥32 to <36 mm (corrected for body size [PSAX/BSA] ≥ 18 to <21 mm/m^2) • O fractional area change >33% to ≤40% By MRI: regional RV akinesia or dyskinesia or dyssynchronous RV contraction and one of the following: • Ratio of RV end-diastolic volume to BSA ≥ 100 to <110 mL/m^2 (male) or ≥90 to <100 mL/m^2 (female) • RV ejection fraction >40% to ≤45%
II. Tissue characterization of the wall	
Major	Residual myocytes <60% by morphometric analysis (or <50% if estimated), with fibrous replacement of the RV free wall myocardium in ≥1 sample, with or without fatty replacement of tissue on endomyocardial biopsy
Minor	Residual myocytes 60% to 75% by morphometric analysis (or 50% to 65% if estimated), with fibrous replacement of the RV free wall myocardium in ≥1 sample, with or without fatty replacement of tissue on endomyocardial biopsy
II. Repolarization abnormalities	
Major	Epsilon wave (reproducible low-amplitude signals between the end of QRS complex to onset of the T wave) in the right precordial leads (V1 to V3)
Minor	Late potentials by SAECG in ≥1 of 3 parameters in the absence of a QRS duration of ≥110 ms on the standard ECG: filtered QRS duration (fQRS) ≥ 114 ms; duration of terminal QRS < 40 μV (low-amplitude signal duration) ≥ 38 ms; root-mean-square voltage of terminal 40 ms ≤ 20μV. Terminal activation duration of QRS ≥ 55 ms measured from the nadir of the S wave to the end of the QRS, including R', in V1, V2 or V3, in the absence of complete RBBB
V. Arrhythmias	
Major	Nonsustained or sustained ventricular tachycardia of left bundle-branch morphology with superior axis (negative or indeterminate QRS in leads II, III and aVF and positive in lead aVL)
Minor	Nonsustained or sustained ventricular tachycardia of RVOT configuration, LBBB morphology with inferior axis (positive QRS in leads II, III and aVF and negative in lead aVL) or of unknown axis > 500 ventricular extrasystoles per 24 h (Holter)
VI. Family history	
Major	ARVC/D confirmed in a first-degree relative who meets current Task Force criteria ARVC/D confirmed pathologically at autopsy or surgery in a first-degree relative. Identification of a pathogenic mutation * categorized as associated or probably associated with ARVC/D in the patient under evaluation
Minor	History of ARVC/D in a first-degree relative in whom it is not possible or practical to determine whether the family member meets current Task Force criteria. Premature sudden death (<35 years of age) due to suspected ARVC/D in a first-degree relative. ARVC/D confirmed pathologically or by current Task Force criteria in second-degree relative

Definite diagnosis: two major criteria or one major and two minor criteria. Borderline diagnosis: one major and two minor. Possible diagnosis: one major or two minor criteria

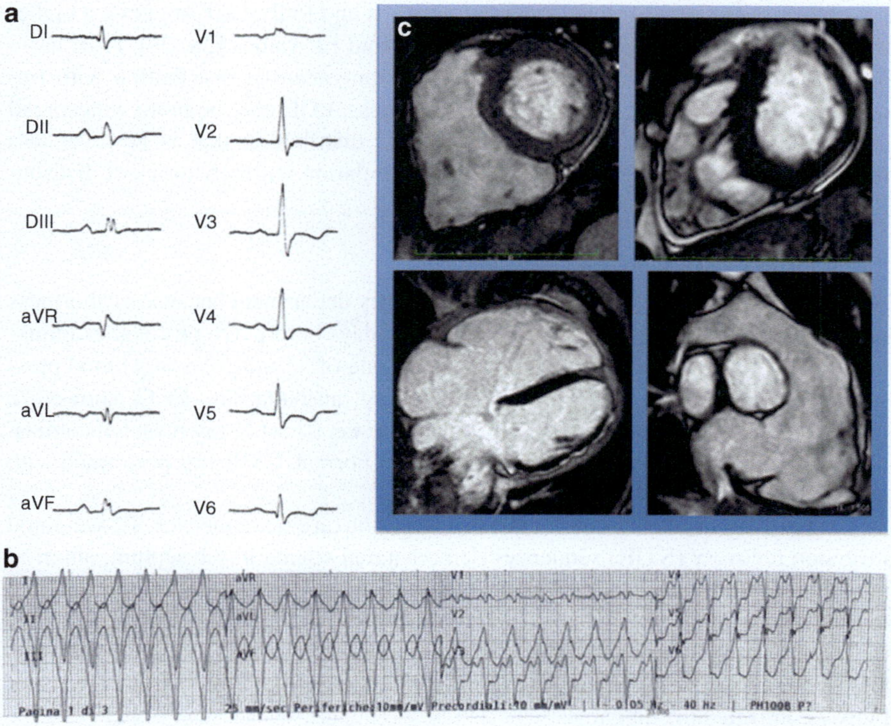

Fig. 5.10 A case of ARVC with ECG findings (panel **a**), TV from the RB (BBS morphology with superior axis in panel **b**) and CMR evidence of segmental and global RV dysfunction (panel **c**) consistent with the clinical diagnosis

(panel a), previous recording of VT with LBB morphology and superior axis (panel b) and CMR findings with RV dilatation (telediastolic RV volume is >110 mL/m2, RVEF is <40%) and RVOT dilatation and dyskinesia as evidence of ARVC (panel c).

5.4 Inflammatory Cardiomyopathies

Such subgroup mainly includes sarcoidosis and CMPs associated with systemic inflammatory diseases.

5.4.1 Sarcoidosis

Sarcoidosis is a granulomatous inflammatory disease with multi-organ involvement that may affect the heart. A symptomatic cardiac involvement is documented in 5% of cases but can be confirmed in 25% by autopsy and in 20% of patients by CMR: on this basis, CMR is suggested as a diagnostic test to confirm cardiac involvement in sarcoidosis [1, 27]. In the presence of sarcoidosis with cardiac involvement, it is possible to detect myocardial edema, myocarditis and LGE. LGE suggests a higher risk of arrhythmias and death, independently from EF values [28, 29]. LGE has a non-ischemic pattern with subepicardial or intramyocardial distribution with frequent involvement of the lateral wall. Nevertheless, LGE may be more widespread and even have a transmural or subendocardial distribution that is however less intense than in ischemic forms and without correlation with territories of distribution of coronary arteries.

5.4.1.1 Case with Sarcoidosis

A 46-year-old man was admitted to the emergency department because of shortness of breath and fainting. He suffered syncope few days before. On physical examination, he demonstrated bradycardia with a heart rate of 35/min, elevated blood pressure (160/90 mmHg) and normal pulmonary auscultation. ECG showed a third-degree AV block with a wide QRS of 140 msec. Chest X-ray revealed mediastinal lymphadenopathies. Echocardiography was normal. CMR was performed with the clinical suspicion of sarcoidosis.

Cardiac MR revealed normal ventricular function on cine sequences. T2-weighted inversion recovery (STIR) sequences demonstrated edema in the septum, anterior, anterolateral and inferior wall (Fig. 5.11: see red arrows) with non-ischemic LGE in the same LV segments (Fig. 5.11: see white arrows). In conclusion, CMR confirmed the clinical suspicion of sarcoidosis with cardiac involvement. Chest CT-scan was also performed showing interstitial nodules (5 mm diameter), and a trans-bronchial biopsy confirmed the diagnosis.

5.4.2 Cardiomyopathies Associated with Systemic Inflammatory Diseases

In the setting of systemic inflammatory diseases (e.g. SLE, rheumatoid arthritis, vasculitis), cardiovascular involvement can be detected by CMR in different forms: accelerated atherosclerosis with perfusion defects and ischemic scars, myocarditis, pericarditis, heart valve diseases and vasculitis [1].

5.5 Infiltrative Cardiomyopathies (Amyloidosis, Hemochromatosis, Anderson-Fabry Disease)

In the setting of infiltrative CMP, CMR allows a more precise evaluation of segmental and global biventricular function coupled with the possibility of tissue characterization of the infiltration (Table 5.4).

In amyloidosis, SSFP images may detect morphological features (ventricular thickening, especially of the interventricular septum, interatrial septum thickening usually >6 mm in 20% of cases, biatrial dilatation and the presence of pericardial and pleural effusions). On LGE imaging, the typical finding is that it is difficult to assess the optimal inversion time on scout sequences since amyloid has high affinity

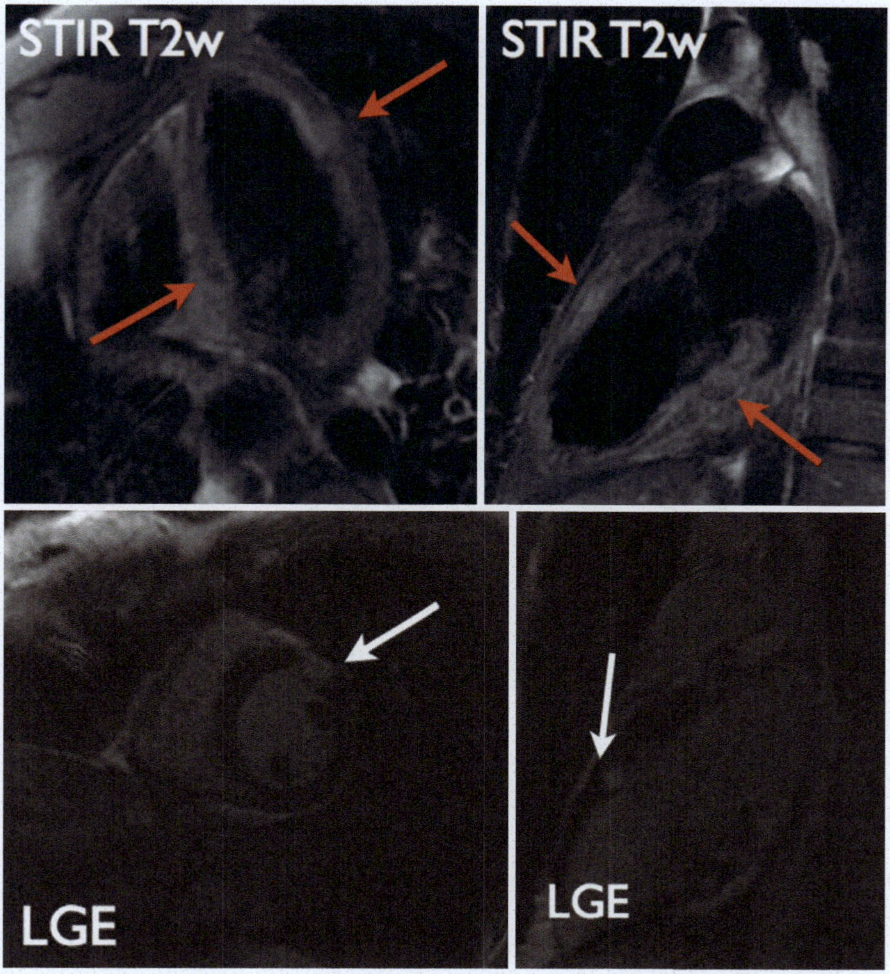

Fig. 5.11 A case with cardiac sarcoidosis and evidence of myocardial edema (see red arrows) and non-ischemic LGE in the same segments (see white arrows)

Table 5.4 CMR and infiltrative CMP

Infiltrative CMP	Pathological substance	CMR findings
Amyloidosis	AL amyloidosis Transthyretin amyloidosis (ATTR)	Wall thickness, biatrial dilatation, subendocardial LGE
Hemochromatosis	Iron	Reduced T2* proportional to the degree of iron overload
Anderson-Fabry disease	Glycosphingolipids	LV wall thickening with non-ischemic LGE in 50% of cases (usually subepicardial inferolateral). Being an accumulation of lipids, native T1 is reduced in the pathological tissue

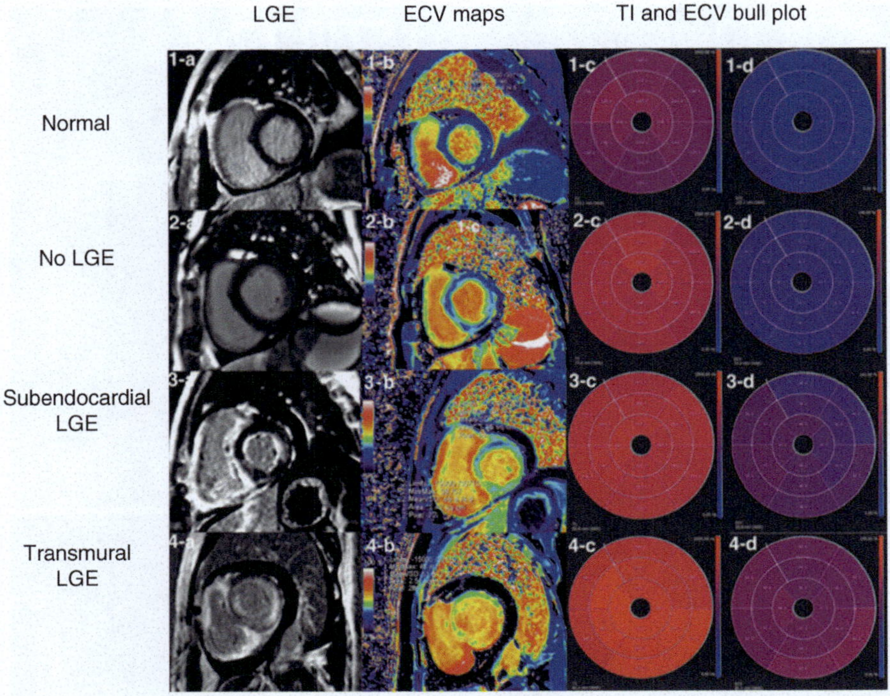

Fig. 5.12 Cases with increasing degrees of LGE in amyloidosis: (**a**) normal case, (**b**) a case of amyloidosis without significant LGE, (**c**) subendocardial LGE and (**d**) extensive transmural LGE. T1 and ECV are progressively increased with more extensive infiltration and LGE. From Lin L. et al. J Cardiovasc Magn Reson. 2018 Jan 3;20(1):2

for the contrast medium. LGE is typically more or less extensive usually subendocardial but even transmural in more advanced forms (Fig. 5.12) [30, 31].

According to LGE, it has been proposed a score for the differentiation of AL amyloidosis and ATTR (ATTR = Amyloidosis Transthyretin-Related). The QUALE (Query Amyloid Late Enhancement) score is based on the extent of LGE. In ATTR it is more frequently transmural (around 90% of cases) and involves the right ventricle more commonly than AL [32]. The QUALE score (Fig. 5.13) uses three sections of the ventricles (basal, mid and apical) with a score to be given for each section from 0 (=no LGE) to 4 (circumferential and transmural LGE) till a maximum score of 12. If RV involvement is present, it should be added 6 and thus the maximum score is 18. A score ≥13 is able to differentiate ATTR from AL with a sensitivity of 82% and specificity of 76% [32].

Despite a more extensive LGE in ATTR, its prognosis is better than AL because of a different availability and efficacy of treatments (Table 5.5).

Anderson-Fabry disease is a genetically determined X-linked disease that affects the metabolism of glycosphingolipids, and it is characterized by accumulation of these metabolitis in endothelial cells with possible ischemia and infarcts involving

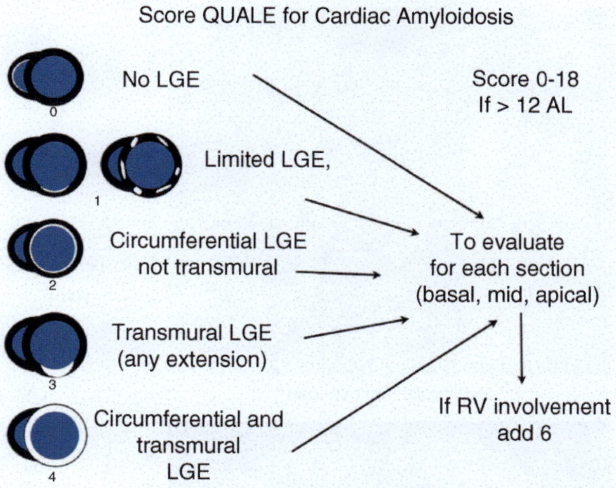

Fig. 5.13 QUALE score for the evaluation of amyloidosis according to LGE extension

Table 5.5 Differential diagnosis between ATTR and AL

Feature	ATTR	AL
LV mass	Markedly increased (>100 g/m^2)	Increased (<100 g/m^2)
IVS thickness	++	+
Native T1 (mapping)	$T1_{AL}$ > 1050–1150 ms > $T1_{ATTR}$	
LGE	Extensive	Less extensive
Therapy	New specific therapies	Chemotherapy
Prognosis	Better	Worse

different tissues and organs. The heart, kidney, brain and skin are especially affected with different symptoms including pain at the extremities (acroparesthesia), neuropathic pain, headache, kidney insufficiency and heart disease with accumulation of lipids. In CMR, it is possible to detect the thickening of LV with LGE that is typically subepicardial and involving the inferolateral wall. Since it is a pathological accumulation of lipids, native T1 values are reduced in areas with lipid accumulation (Fig. 5.2); however T1 values may be increased in areas with replacement fibrosis [33, 34].

Hemochromatosis is characterized by the pathological accumulation of iron that may affect the heart and liver. CMR can identify and quantify the iron overload in both organs by the estimation of T2* that is progressively reduced with increasing levels of iron in tissues. Gradient-echo sequences allow the calculation of tissue T2* in the heart and liver by selection of a region of interest (usually in the interventricular septum in the heart) [35, 36]. A case example is reported in Fig. 5.14 with both heart and liver iron overload. Hemochromatosis may be primary (genetic disease) or secondary to iron overload following repeated blood transfusions (e.g. thalassemia or myelodysplastic diseases). Diagnostic values of T2* are reported in Table 5.6.

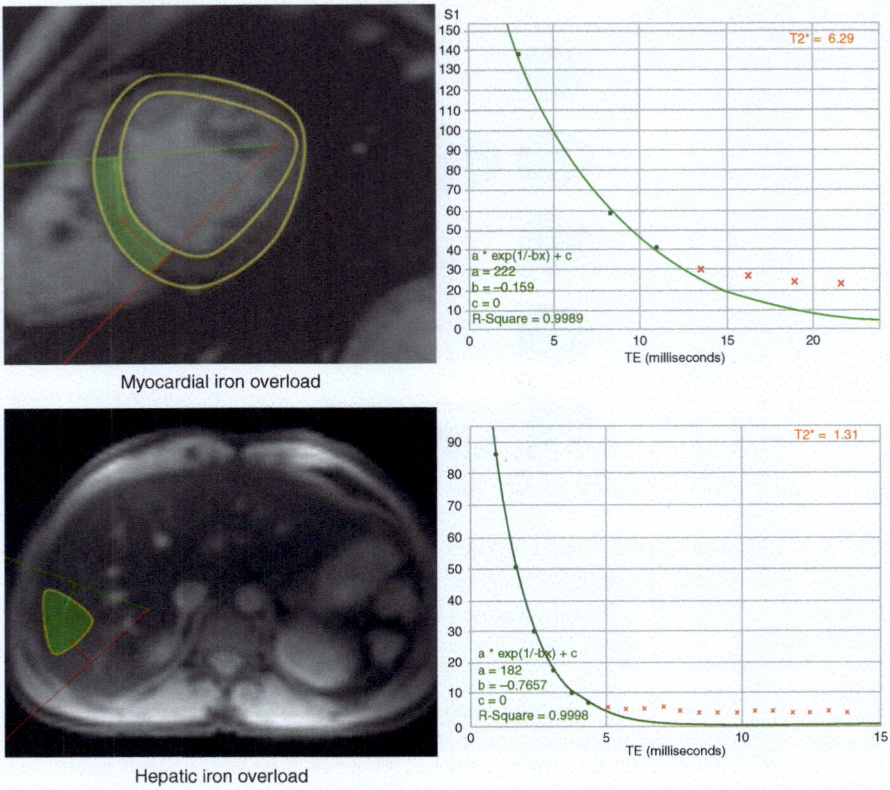

Fig. 5.14 A case with heart and liver iron overload. Gradient-echo sequences allow the estimation of T2* that is 6.29 in the heart (see septal region of interest in green) and liver with a value of 1.31 (see hepatic region of interest in green). From Garbowski et al. Journal of Cardiovascular Magnetic Resonance 2014, 16:40. Open access (per sovraccario epatico)

Table 5.6 Diagnostic values of T2* for the diagnosis and grading of iron overload

Myocardial T2* (ms)	Degree of iron overload
≥20	Absent
14–20	Mild
10–14	Moderate
≤10	Severe
Hepatic T2* (ms)	Degree of iron overload
≥15.4	Absent
4.5–15.4	Mild
2.1–4.5	Moderate
≤2.1	Severe

5.6 Takotsubo Syndrome

Takotsubo syndrome has been described for the first time by Sato et al. in 1990. The name is derived from the typical Japanese octopus trap and recalls the morphology of a dilated akinetic apex of the LV affected by the syndrome [37–39] (Fig. 5.15).

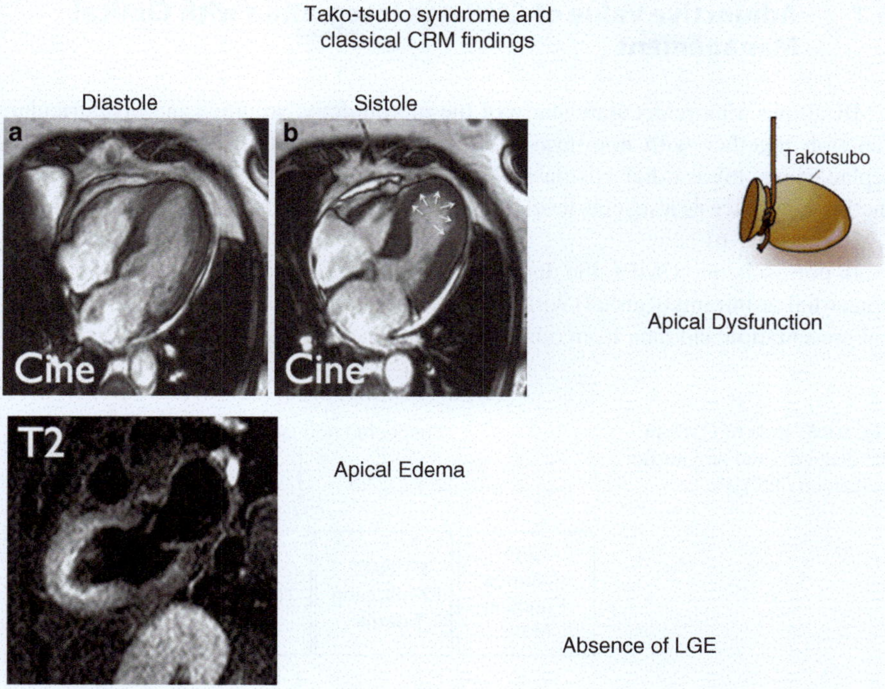

Fig. 5.15 A typical case with Takotsubo syndrome: apical ballooning with apical akinesia (panels **a**, **b**), edema (T2w) and the absence of LGE in affected segments. Modified from Plácido et al. Journal of Cardiovascular Magnetic Resonance (2016) 18:68. Open access

The pathophysiology of Takotsubo syndrome is similar to that of an acute coronary syndrome triggered by stress in a predisposed subject with microcirculation dysfunction [39], rather than a cardiomyopathy. The typical patient is a woman in postmenopausal age after a physical or emotional stress. The recovery starts after few days and it is usually complete after few weeks. CMR allows to confirm the diagnosis and exclude other possible conditions to be considered in the differential diagnosis (e.g. myocardial infarction and myocarditis) [34, 35].

Peculiar CMR findings in Takotsubo syndrome [34, 35] include:

1. Apical dysfunction with apical akinesia and hyperkinesia of basal segments
2. Apical edema on T2w imaging (affects the same segments with dysfunction)
3. Absence of LGE in affected segments
4. Reversibility during follow-up after 3–6 months from the initial presentation

The usual CMR protocol for the evaluation of Takotsubo syndrome includes cine SSFP (study of kinesis and function), STIR T2w imaging (study of myocardial edema) and LGE.

An illustrative case is reported in Fig. 5.13.

5.7 Adjunctive Value of CMR and Integration with Clinical Management

CMR allows a more accurate study of the morphology, volumes and biventricular function together with non-invasive tissue characterization (study of fibro-fatty replacement, myocardial edema and scars). On this basis, CMR is the imaging method of choice as a second-level imaging test for the study of suspected or known CMPs (Fig. 5.16).

In non-ischemic CMPs, the distribution of LGE is typically non-ischemic (subepicardial or intramyocardial) with non-specific features to be correlated with clinical presentation and data from other CMR sequences (Fig. 5.17).

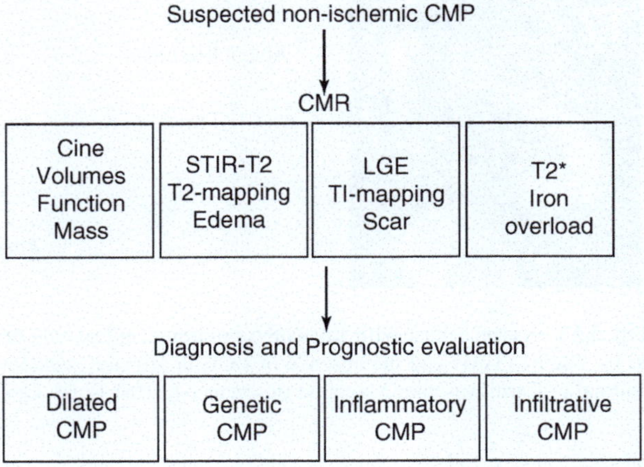

Fig. 5.16 Role of CMR in the diagnosis and prognostic evaluation of CMPs

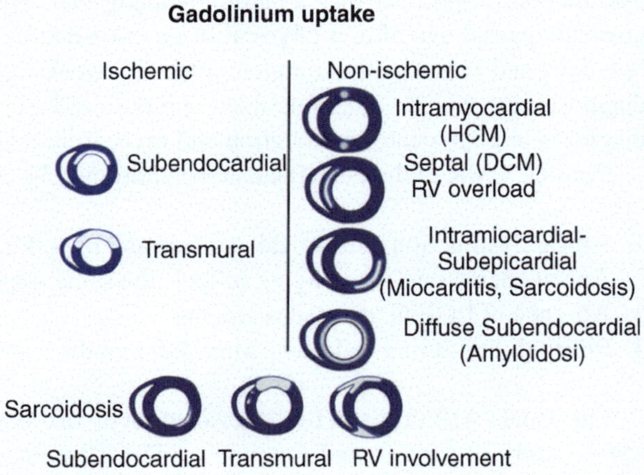

Fig. 5.17 Ischemic and non-ischemic LGE. In sarcoidosis and amyloidosis, LGE may have different patterns of distribution that may sometimes mimic ischemic patterns (subendocardial and transmural) but without correspondence with territories of distribution of coronary arteries

Table 5.7 Standard CMR protocol for the evaluation of a suspected or known CMP

Sequence	Derived data
Cine	Morphology, volumes and biventricular function
T1w imaging (with and without fat saturation)	Morphology and study of fibro-fatty replacement
Native T1	Evaluation of interstitial and infiltrative processes
STIR T2w	Evaluation of myocardial edema
T2*	Evaluation of iron overload
LGE	Evaluation of distribution and entity of myocardial scars

LGE late gadolinium enhancement

5.8 Key Points and Protocols

- CMR is the gold standard for the evaluation of volumes and biventricular function; moreover it allows a good morphological evaluation and non-invasive tissue characterization. On this basis, CMPs are one of the main indications of CMR.
- The standard CMR protocol for the study of CMPs includes cine sequences, T1w imaging (with and without fat suppression), T2w imaging, T1 mapping (if available), T2* evaluation for iron overload, EGE (if thrombi should be excluded) and LGE (Table 5.7).
- Native T1 mapping may allow to identify diffuse processes but also specific forms (e.g. low values of T1 for fat, iron overload and Anderson-Fabry disease, high values for myocarditis and amyloidosis) without the use of contrast agents.

References

1. Patel AR, Kramer CM. Role of cardiac magnetic resonance in the diagnosis and prognosis of nonischemic cardiomyopathy. JACC Cardiovasc Imaging. 2017;10(10 Pt A):1180–93.
2. Bruder O, Wagner A, Lombardi M, Schwitter J, van Rossum A, Pilz G, Nothnagelv D, Steen H, Petersen S, Nagel E, Prasad S, Schumm J, Greulich S, Cagnolo A, Monney P, Deluigi CC, Dill T, Frank H, Sabin G, Schneider S, Mahrholdt H. European Cardiovascular Magnetic Resonance (EuroCMR) registry – multi national results from 57 centers in 15 countries. J Cardiovasc Magn Reson. 2013;15:9. https://doi.org/10.1186/1532-429X-15-9.
3. Aquaro GD, Di Bella G, Castelletti S, et al. Clinical recommendation of cardiac magnetic resonance, part II: inflammatory and congenital heart disease, cardiomyopathies and cardiac tumors: a position paper of the working group "Applicazioni della Risonanza Magnetica" of the Italian Society of Cardiology. J Cardiovasc Med. 2017;18:209–22.
4. Gulati A, Jabbour A, Ismail TF, Guha K, Khwaja J, Raza S, Morarji K, Brown TD, Ismail NA, Dweck MR, Di Pietro E, Roughton M, Wage R, Daryani Y, O'Hanlon R, Sheppard MN, Alpendurada F, Lyon AR, Cook SA, Cowie MR, Assomull RG, Pennell DJ, Prasad SK. Association of fibrosis with mortality and sudden cardiac death in patients with nonischemic dilated cardiomyopathy. JAMA. 2013;309(9):896–908.

5. Mikami Y, Cornhill A, Heydari B, Joncas SX, Almehmadi F, Zahrani M, Bokhari M, Stirrat J, Yee R, Merchant N, Lydell CP, Howarth AG, White JA. Objective criteria for septal fibrosis in non-ischemic dilated cardiomyopathy: validation for the prediction of future cardiovascular events. J Cardiovasc Magn Reson. 2016;18(1):82.
6. Messroghli DR, Moon JC, Ferreira VM, Grosse-Wortmann L, He T, Kellman P, Mascherbauer J, Nezafat R, Salerno M, Schelbert EB, Taylor AJ, Thompson R, Ugander M, van Heeswijk RB. Friedrich MG. Clinical recommendations for cardiovascular magnetic resonance mapping of T1, T2, T2* and extracellular volume: a consensus statement by the Society for Cardiovascular Magnetic Resonance (SCMR) endorsed by the European Association for Cardiovascular Imaging (EACVI). J Cardiovasc Magn Reson. 2017;19(1):75.
7. Semsarian C, Ingles J, Maron MS, Maron BJ. New perspectives on the prevalence of hypertrophic cardiomyopathy. J Am Coll Cardiol. 2015;65(12):1249–54.
8. Authors/Task Force Members, Elliott PM, Anastasakis A, Borger MA, Borggrefe M, Cecchi F, Charron P, Hagege AA, Lafont A, Limongelli G, Mahrholdt H, WJ MK, Mogensen J, Nihoyannopoulos P, Nistri S, Pieper PG, Pieske B, Rapezzi C, Rutten FH, Tillmanns C. 2014 ESC Guidelines on diagnosis and management of hypertrophic cardiomyopathy: the Task Force for the Diagnosis and Management of Hypertrophic Cardiomyopathy of the European Society of Cardiology (ESC). Eur Heart J. 2014;35(39):2733–79.
9. Noureldin RA, Liu S, Nacif MS, Judge DP, Halushka MK, Abraham TP, Ho C, Bluemke DA. The diagnosis of hypertrophic cardiomyopathy by cardiovascular magnetic resonance. J Cardiovasc Magn Reson. 2012;14:17.
10. Maron MS. Clinical utility of cardiovascular magnetic resonance in hypertrophic cardiomyopathy. J Cardiovasc Magn Reson. 2012;14(1):13.
11. Hindieh W, Chan R, Rakowski H. Complementary role of echocardiography and cardiac magnetic resonance in hypertrophic cardiomyopathy. Curr Cardiol Rep. 2017;19(9):81.
12. Choudhury L, Rigolin VH, Bonow RO. Integrated imaging in hypertrophic cardiomyopathy. Am J Cardiol. 2017;119(2):328–39.
13. Marchesini M, Uguccioni L, Parisi R, Mattioli G, Terzi F, Olivieri R, Capucci A, Fattori R. The role of cardiac magnetic resonance imaging in hypertrophic cardiomyopathy. Rev Cardiovasc Med. 2016;17(1–2):57–64.
14. Child N, Muhr T, Sammut E, Dabir D, Ucar EA, Bueser T, Gill J, Carr-White G, Nagel E, Puntmann VO. Prevalence of myocardial crypts in a large retrospective cohort study by cardiovascular magnetic resonance. J Cardiovasc Magn Reson. 2014;16:66.
15. Weng Z, Yao J, Chan RH, He J, Yang X, Zhou Y, He Y. Prognostic value of LGE-CMR in HCM: a meta-analysis. JACC Cardiovasc Imaging. 2016;9(12):1392–402.
16. Towbin JA, Lorts A, Jefferies JL. Left ventricular non-compaction cardiomyopathy. Lancet. 2015;386(9995):813–25.
17. Elliott P, Andersson B, Arbustini E, Bilinska Z, Cecchi F, Charron P, Dubourg O, Kühl U, Maisch B, McKenna WJ, Monserrat L, Pankuweit S, Rapezzi C, Seferovic P, Tavazzi L, Keren A. Classification of the cardiomyopathies: a position statement from the European Society of Cardiology Working Group on Myocardial and Pericardial Diseases. Eur Heart J. 2008;29(2):270–6.
18. Zemrak F, Ahlman MA, Captur G, Mohiddin SA, Kawel-Boehm N, Prince MR, Moon JC, Hundley WG, Lima JA, Bluemke DA, Petersen SE. The relationship of left ventricular trabeculation to ventricular function and structure over a 9.5-year follow-up: the MESA study. J Am Coll Cardiol. 2014;64(19):1971–80.
19. Jenni R, Wyss CA, Oechslin EN, Kaufmann PA. Isolated ventricular noncompaction is associated with coronary microcirculatory dysfunction. J Am Coll Cardiol. 2002;39(3):450–4.
20. Petersen SE, Selvanayagam JB, Wiesmann F, Robson MD, Francis JM, Anderson RH, Watkins H, Neubauer S. Left ventricular non-compaction: insights from cardiovascular magnetic resonance imaging. J Am Coll Cardiol. 2005;46(1):101–5.
21. Jacquier A, Thuny F, Jop B, Giorgi R, Cohen F, Gaubert JY, Vidal V, Bartoli JM, Habib G, Moulin G. Measurement of trabeculated left ventricular mass using cardiac magnetic resonance imaging in the diagnosis of left ventricular non-compaction. Eur Heart J. 2010;31(9):1098–104.

22. Stacey RB, Andersen MM, St Clair M, Hundley WG, Thohan V. Comparison of systolic and diastolic criteria for isolated LV noncompaction in CMR. JACC Cardiovasc Imaging. 2013;6(9):931–40.
23. Caselli S, Ferreira D, Kanawati E, Di Paolo F, Pisicchio C, Attenhofer Jost C, Spataro A, Jenni R, Pelliccia A. Prominent left ventricular trabeculations in competitive athletes: a proposal for risk stratification and management. Int J Cardiol. 2016;223:590–5.
24. Marcus FI, McKenna WJ, Sherrill D, Basso C, Bauce B, Bluemke DA, Calkins H, Corrado D, Cox MG, Daubert JP, Fontaine G, Gear K, Hauer R, Nava A, Picard MH, Protonotarios N, Saffitz JE, Sanborn DM, Steinberg JS, Tandri H, Thiene G, Towbin JA, Tsatsopoulou A, Wichter T, Zareba W. Diagnosis of arrhythmogenic right ventricular cardiomyopathy/dysplasia: proposed modification of the Task Force Criteria. Eur Heart J. 2010;31(7): 806–14.
25. Vermes E, Strohm O, Otmani A, Childs H, Duff H, Friedrich MG. Impact of the revision of arrhythmogenic right ventricular cardiomyopathy/dysplasia task force criteria on its prevalence by CMR criteria. JACC Cardiovasc Imaging. 2011;4(3):282–7.
26. Haugaa KH, Basso C, Badano LP, Bucciarelli-Ducci C, Cardim N, Gaemperli O, Galderisi M, Habib G, Knuuti J, Lancellotti P, McKenna W, Neglia D, Popescu BA, Edvardsen T, EACVI Scientific Documents Committee, EACVI Board members and external reviewers; EACVI Scientific Documents Committee, EACVI Board Members and External Reviewers. Comprehensive multi-modality imaging approach in arrhythmogenic cardiomyopathy-an expert consensus document of the European Association of Cardiovascular Imaging. Eur Heart J Cardiovasc Imaging. 2017;18(3):237–53.
27. Writing Group; Document Reading Group; EACVI Reviewers: This document was reviewed by members of the EACVI Scientific Documents Committee for 2014–2016 and 2016–2018. A joint procedural position statement on imaging in cardiac sarcoidosis: from the Cardiovascular and Inflammation & Infection Committees of the European Association of Nuclear Medicine, the European Association of Cardiovascular Imaging, and the American Society of Nuclear Cardiology. Eur Heart J Cardiovasc Imaging. 2017;18(10):1073–89.
28. Hulten E, Agarwal V, Cahill M, Cole G, Vita T, Parrish S, Bittencourt MS, Murthy VL, Kwong R, Di Carli MF, Blankstein R. Presence of late gadolinium enhancement by cardiac magnetic resonance among patients with suspected cardiac sarcoidosis is associated with adverse cardiovascular prognosis: a systematic review and meta-analysis. Circ Cardiovasc Imaging. 2016;9(9):e005001. https://doi.org/10.1161/CIRCIMAGING.116.005001.
29. Coleman GC, Shaw PW, Balfour PC Jr, Gonzalez JA, Kramer CM, Patel AR, Salerno M. Prognostic value of myocardial scarring on CMR in patients with cardiac sarcoidosis. JACC Cardiovasc Imaging. 2017;10(4):411–20.
30. Habib G, Bucciarelli-Ducci C, ALP C, Cardim N, Charron P, Cosyns B, Dehaene A, Derumeaux G, Donal E, Dweck MR, Edvardsen T, Erba PA, Ernande L, Gaemperli O, Galderisi M, Grapsa J, Jacquier A, Klingel K, Lancellotti P, Neglia D, Pepe A, Perrone-Filardi P, Petersen SE, Plein S, Popescu BA, Reant P, Sade LE, Salaun E, RHJA S, Tribouilloy C, Zamorano J, EACVI Scientific Documents Committee; Indian Academy of Echocardiography. Multimodality imaging in restrictive cardiomyopathies: an EACVI expert consensus document in collaboration with the "Working Group on myocardial and pericardial diseases" of the European Society of Cardiology Endorsed by The Indian Academy of Echocardiography. Eur Heart J Cardiovasc Imaging. 2017;18(10):1090–121.
31. Lin L, Li X, Feng J, Shen KN, Tian Z, Sun J, Mao YY, Cao J, Jin ZY, Li J, Selvanayagam JB, Wang YN. The prognostic value of T1 mapping and late gadolinium enhancement cardiovascular magnetic resonance imaging in patients with light chain amyloidosis. J Cardiovasc Magn Reson. 2018;20(1):2.
32. Dungu JN, Valencia O, Pinney JH, et al. CMR-based differentiation of AL and ATTR cardiac amyloidosis. JACC Cardiovasc Imaging. 2014;7(2):133–42.
33. Hoigné P, Attenhofer Jost CH, Duru F, et al. Simple criteria for differentiation of Fabry disease from amyloid heart disease and other causes of left ventricular hypertrophy. Int J Cardiol. 2006;111(3):413–22.

34. Sado DM, White SK, Piechnik SK, et al. Identification and assessment of Anderson-Fabry disease by cardiovascular magnetic resonance noncontrast myocardial T1 mapping. Circ Cardiovasc Imaging. 2013;6(3):392–8.
35. Smith GC, Carpenter JP, He T, Alam MH, Firmin DN, Pennell DJ. Value of black blood T2* cardiovascular magnetic resonance. J Cardiovasc Magn Reson. 2011;13:21.
36. Garbowski MW, Carpenter JP, Smith G, Roughton M, Alam MH, He T, Pennell DJ, Porter JB. Biopsy-based calibration of T2* magnetic resonance for estimation of liver iron concentration and comparison with R2 Ferriscan. J Cardiovasc Magn Reson. 2014;16:40.
37. Plácido R, Cunha Lopes B, Almeida AG, Rochitte CE. The role of cardiovascular magnetic resonance in takotsubo syndrome. J Cardiovasc Magn Reson. 2016;18(1):68.
38. Naruse Y, Sato A, Kasahara K, Makino K, Sano M, Takeuchi Y, Nagasaka S, Wakabayashi Y, Katoh H, Satoh H, Hayashi H, Aonuma K. The clinical impact of late gadolinium enhancement in Takotsubo cardiomyopathy: serial analysis of cardiovascular magnetic resonance images. J Cardiovasc Magn Reson. 2011;13:67.
39. Pelliccia F, Sinagra G, Elliott P, Parodi G, Basso C, Camici PG. Takotsubo is not a cardiomyopathy. Int J Cardiol. 2018;254:250–3.

Myocarditis

6

Contents

6.1 Introduction

Myocarditis is an inflammatory disease of the myocardium due to infectious or non-infectious agents. The definite diagnosis of myocarditis is based on endomyocardial biopsy (EMB) with demonstration of inflammation of the myocardium [1]. The etiological spectrum of myocarditis is wide and overlaps with pericarditis (Table 6.1): for this reason pericarditis and myocarditis can coexist in overlapping forms usually named as myopericarditis or perimyocarditis [2–6].

According to 2015 ESC guidelines on the diagnosis and management of pericardial diseases [7], *myopericarditis* is pericarditis with myocarditis and preserved

Table 6.1 Common etiologies of myocarditis and myopericardial inflammatory syndromes

Idiopathic
Infectious
Viral (Coxsackie, adenoviruses, herpes virus, CMV, EBV, VZV, influenza, hepatitis A and C, parvovirus B19)
Bacterial (tuberculosis, *Campylobacter jejuni*, *Neisseria meningitidis*, *Chlamydophila*)
Other (rare)
Non-infectious (usually immune-mediated)
Systemic inflammatory diseases (e.g. gigantocellular arteritis, lupus, Still disease)
Inflammatory bowel disease
Vaccine-related (smallpox, diphtheria, tetanus, poliomyelitis)
Drug-related (5-fluorouracile, phenytoin, clozapine, mesalazine)

M. Imazio et al., *Learning Cardiac Magnetic Resonance*,
https://doi.org/10.1007/978-3-030-11608-8_6

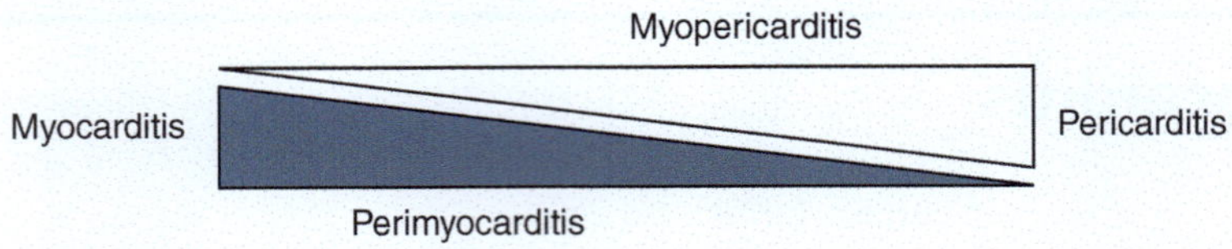

	Pericarditis	Myopericarditis	Perimyocarditis
Pericarditis Criteria	+	+	+
Troponin Elevation	Absent	Usually present	Usually present
EF WMSI	Normal	Normal	Reduced EF WMSI>I

Fig. 6.1 The spectrum of myopericardial inflammatory diseases

biventricular function, while perimyocarditis is myocarditis with pericarditis and evidence of reduced segmental or global ventricular function (Fig. 6.1).

The clinical spectrum is also variable ranging from asymptomatic forms to sudden cardiac death (SCD): myocarditis is a cause of SCD in 12 to 22% of cases of the young in autoptic series [1, 8–10]. Usually, in clinical practice, myocarditis can have three more common presentations:

1. Pseudo-myocardial infection with chest pain mimicking an AMI (most common)
2. Arrhythmias
3. Heart failure

It is more common in young males for hormonal causes [2, 3, 11]. Clinical criteria for the diagnosis of myocarditis require the integration of clinical evaluation, ECG and imaging data up to EBM in complicated cases because of this heterogeneity of clinical presentation. CMR is now a well-established non-invasive tool for the diagnosis of myocarditis being able to detect myocardial edema, hyperemia and fibrosis and allowing, at the same time, a more precise evaluation of biventricular volumes and function [9, 10].

6.2 CMR Criteria for the Diagnosis of Myocarditis

Myocarditis as any other inflammatory process is responsible of the appearance of edema, hyperemia and possible necrosis with fibrosis. CMR may allow to identify each of these components with specific sequences: STIR T2-weighted imaging detects myocardial edema, EGE allows to identify myocardial hyperemia, while the presence of scars may be identified by LGE [9, 10]. To be more precise, the presence of LGE identifies an increased extracellular space that is due to necrosis, edema and fibrosis in the acute phase (up to 3 months) and myocardial scar in the chronic phase as after an acute myocardial infarction.

Specific limitations of CMR in the evaluation of myocarditis [1, 9–12] include:

1. CMR cannot identify the etiological agent but only the tissue changes caused by the inflammatory process.
2. Inflammatory changes have a short time course: if myocarditis is suspected, CMR should be performed within 2 to 4 weeks from symptoms onset in order to detect hyperemia and edema.
3. Availability of CMR is limited, and it is more expensive than other non-invasive tests although it is the only one that allows a non-invasive tissue characterization.
4. Traditional CMR techniques allow the identification of discrete lesions but are not able to detect a diffuse pathological process (e.g. interstitial edema and fibrosis): for this reason traditional CMR has a better diagnostic accuracy for the study of myocarditis mimicking an acute coronary syndrome rather than forms with a more diffuse involvement of the myocardium such as those with heart failure of arrhythmias (in such cases, when available, T1 and T2 mapping techniques may allow a better recognition of these forms) [13–15].

Classical CMR criteria for the diagnosis of myocarditis have been developed in 2009 by a consensus of CMR experts at the Lake Louise resort in Canada, and they are also known, for this reason, as Lake Louise criteria [16]. They are still valid today although if mapping techniques are available they should be included in the routine evaluation of these patients. Lake Louise criteria for myocarditis include:

1. *Myocardial edema* (STIR T2w imaging): ratio between myocardial signal and remote signal from skeletal muscle >2.0
2. *Myocardial hyperemia* (EGE): ratio between myocardial signal and remote signal from skeletal muscle >4.0
3. *Myocardial late gadolinium enhancement (LGE)*: myocardial signal intensity increased by at least 5 SD from remote myocardium

Sensitivity and specificity criteria for these criteria are reported in Table 6.2.

Myocarditis usually affects the myocardium with a patchy pattern with a non-ischemic distribution (usually subepicardial but also intramyocardial) without correspondence with a specific territory of coronary distribution (Fig. 6.2).

Table 6.2 Sensitivity and specificity of Lake Louise criteria for the diagnosis of myocarditis

Criterion	Sequence	Quantitative data	Sensitivity (%)	Specificity (%)
Edema	STIR T2w	T2 SI > 2.0	70	71
Hyperemia	EGE	EGE ratio > 4.0	74	83
Fibrosis	LGE	LGE > 5 SD[a]	59	86

EGE early gadolinium enhancement, *LGE* late gadolinium enhancement, *SI* signal intensity
[a]SD is for standard deviation

Fig. 6.2 Non-ischemic pattern of LGE in myocarditis compared with ischemic LGE (subendocardial or transmural distribution)

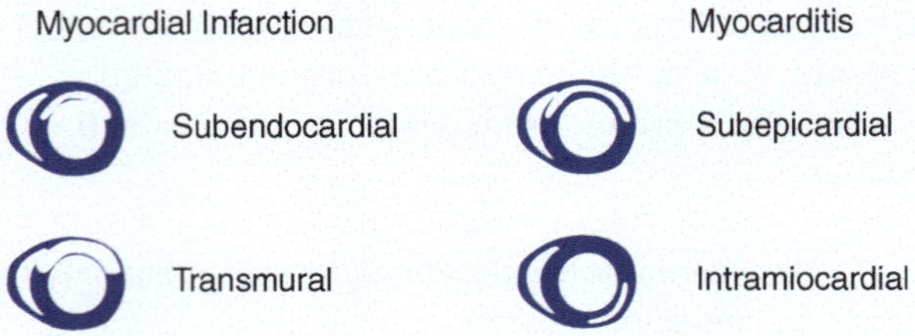

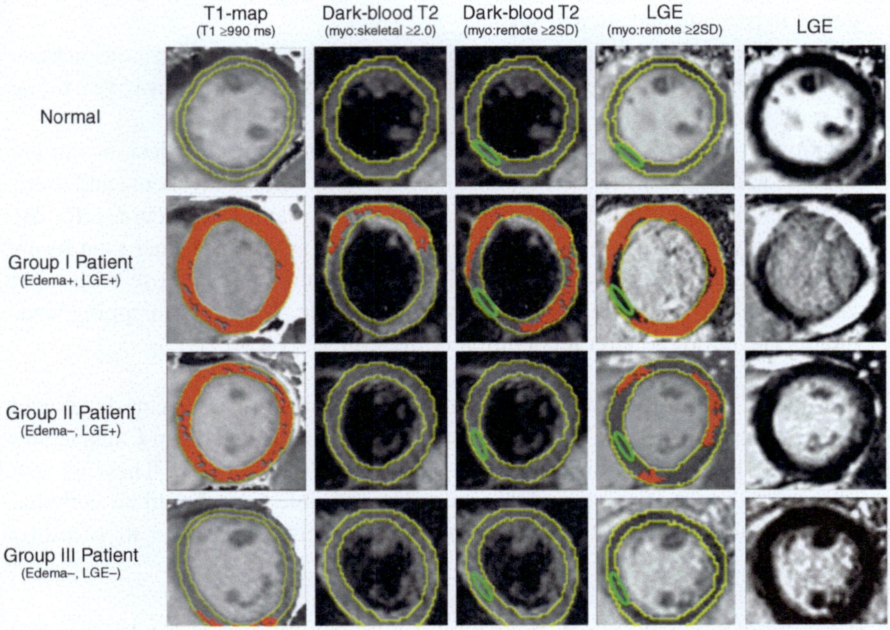

Fig. 6.3 Multiparametric evaluation of cases with acute myocarditis by the use of T1 mapping, dark blood T2 and LGE: a native myocardial T1 > 990 msec identifies larger areas with myocarditis. From Ferreira et al., native T1 mapping detects the location, extent and patterns of acute myocarditis without the need for gadolinium contrast agents. Journal of Cardiovascular Magnetic Resonance 2014 16:36 (open access)

T1 mapping technique allows to assess the value of native myocardial T1 without contrast injection (Fig. 6.3). In the presence of a diffuse interstitial involvement with edema and/or fibrosis, T1 values are increased and may predict the presence of myocarditis with a sensitivity up to 90% compared with traditional techniques (Lake Louise criteria). A value of native myocardial T1 > 990 msec identifies areas with myocarditis with a higher sensitivity and specificity (respectively, 90% and 88%) compared with traditional Lake Louise criteria and without the use of contrast agents [14].

Fig. 6.4 Clinical flow chart for the evaluation of a clinically suspected uncomplicated myocarditis

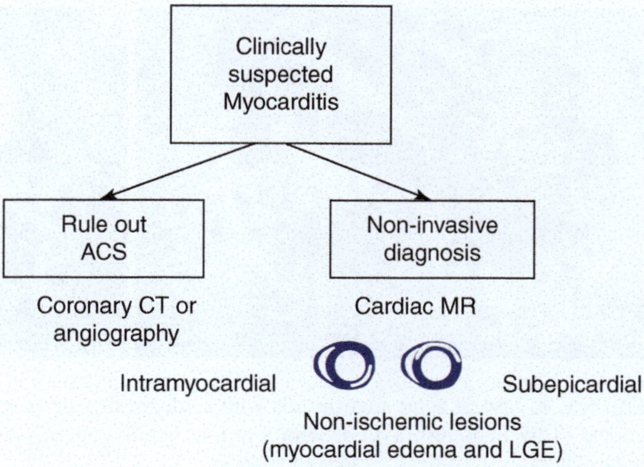

6.3 What Is the Added Value of CMR in the Evaluation of a Patient with Myocarditis

CMR allows the non-invasive diagnosis of myocarditis [16–20] in the setting of uncomplicated myocarditis (usually patients with a presentation with chest pain and preserved biventricular function). In such patients, the course is usually benign, and there is no clinical justification to undergo invasive evaluation for the precise assessment of the etiology since there are no proven specific therapies to offer to this subgroup of patients, at least in clinical practice. In patients with coronary risk factors and a presentation mimicking ischemic chest pain, it is mandatory to rule out an acute coronary syndrome (Fig. 6.4).

On the contrary, patients with complicated myocarditis (e.g. arrhythmias, heart failure or persistent and worsening ventricular dysfunction) should be considered for EBM beyond CMR. These patients have commonly a reduced ventricular function and a more diffuse myocardial involvement that is better detected by T1 mapping methods rather than conventional Lake Louise criteria.

In clinical practice, considering an unselected population, most cases have a presentation with chest pain, preserved ventricular function and uncomplicated course with a good prognosis. Of course, tertiary referral centres and cardiac transplantation centres will recruit more complicated forms, and in these cases, EBM may be required according to clinical judgement.

6.4 Case: Acute Myocarditis with Pseudo-infarct Presentation

Case presentation: A 40-year-old man was admitted for atypical chest pain. On medical history he had no previous relevant diseases but a flu-like syndrome 2 weeks before.

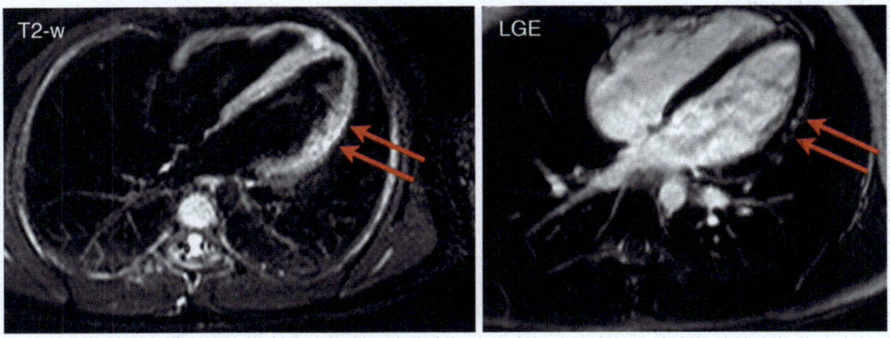

Fig. 6.5 A case of acute myocarditis with evidence of patchy myocardial involvement either as edema (T2w imaging) or LGE with a non-ischemic pattern (subepicardial) at mid-level of the anterolateral wall of the LV (see red arrows)

He complained retrosternal chest pain in two episodes with no relationship with effort and respiration. Chest pain was associated with palpitations and followed by weakness. ECG showed ST segment elevation with isodiphasic T waves on V5–V6, normal CRP and mild elevation of troponin. The patients had no coronary risk factors and were submitted to a CMR study.

CMR findings: A CMR study was performed with cine, T2w imaging, EGE and LGE. Biventricular volumes and function were normal. On T2w imaging, myocardial edema was evident in mid-anterolateral wall as well as patchy subepicardial LGE with non-ischemic pattern suggestive for acute myocarditis according to Lake Louise criteria (Fig. 6.5).

Conclusions: CMR is suggestive for acute myocarditis with preserved biventricular function. Since myocarditis was uncomplicated and associated with preserved ventricular function, the patient was managed conservatively without EBM with medical therapy and was discharged after 1 week after normalization of troponin levels with a planned clinical and echocardiographic follow-up at 6, 12 and 24 months.

6.5 Key Points and CMR Protocol

- In physiological conditions, the normal myocardium does not show edema or late increased signal intensity after gadolinium contrast injection.
- Myocarditis is a cause of myocardial edema, hyperemia and necrosis with possible fibrosis.
- Conventional CMR criteria for the diagnosis of myocarditis include the detection of *myocardial edema* by T2-weighted imaging, *myocardial hyperemia* by EGE and *myocardial LGE* as evidence of increased extracellular space (due to necrosis, edema and fibrosis in the acute setting and scar in chronic cases after at least 3 months). At least two of these three criteria should be met for the CMR diagnosis of acute myocarditis.

Table 6.3 CMR protocol for the evaluation of a patient with clinically suspected myocarditis

CMR sequence	Data
Cine	Evaluation of segmental and global biventricular function
T1 mapping	Evaluation of native myocardial T1 that is increased with interstitial edema and fibrosis (>990 msec) in myocarditis
STIR T2-weighted	Evaluation of myocardial edema
EGE	Evaluation of myocardial hyperemia
LGE	Evaluation of necrosis, edema and fibrosis in the acute phase and myocardial scars in chronic phase. Differential diagnosis with ischemic patterns of LGE

EGE early gadolinium enhancement, *LGE* late gadolinium enhancement (LGE)

- If myocarditis is suspected, CMR should be performed within 2 to 4 weeks from symptoms onset to allow identification of inflammatory signs (e.g. myocardial edema and hyperemia).
- In more diffuse cases with myocardial interstitial edema and fibrosis, conventional criteria have a low diagnostic accuracy, and T1 mapping techniques may allow to study native myocardial T1 without the use of contrast media.
- Increased native myocardial T1 > 990 msec allows to identify myocarditis without the use of gadolinium contrast media.
- The complete CMR protocol for the evaluation of a patient with clinically suspected myocarditis include cine sequences, STIR T2-weighted imaging, EGE and LGE. T1 mapping is to be considered if available (Table 6.3).

References

1. Caforio AL, Pankuweit S, Arbustini E, Basso C, Gimeno-Blanes J, Felix SB, Fu M, Heliö T, Heymans S, Jahns R, Klingel K, Linhart A, Maisch B, McKenna W, Mogensen J, Pinto YM, Ristic A, Schultheiss HP, Seggewiss H, Tavazzi L, Thiene G, Yilmaz A, Charron P, Elliott PM, European Society of Cardiology Working Group on Myocardial and Pericardial Diseases. Current state of knowledge on aetiology, diagnosis, management, and therapy of myocarditis: a position statement of the European Society of Cardiology Working Group on Myocardial and Pericardial Diseases. Eur Heart J. 2013;34:2636–48.
2. Imazio M, Trinchero R. Myopericarditis: etiology, management, and prognosis. Int J Cardiol. 2008;127:17–26.
3. Imazio M, Cooper LT. Management of myopericarditis. Expert Rev Cardiovasc Ther. 2013;11(2):193–201.
4. Imazio M, Brucato A, Barbieri A, Ferroni F, Maestroni S, Ligabue G, Chinaglia A, Cumetti D, Della Casa G, Bonomi F, Mantovani F, Di Corato P, Lugli R, Faletti R, Leuzzi S, Bonamini R, Modena MG, Belli R. Good prognosis for pericarditis with and without myocardial involvement: results from a multicenter, prospective cohort study. Circulation. 2013;128(1):42–9.
5. Imazio M. Le malattie del pericardio. Il Pensiero Scientifico Editore; 2016.
6. Imazio M. Myopericardial diseases. Springer; 2016.
7. Adler Y, Charron P, Imazio M, et al; European Society of Cardiology (ESC). 2015 ESC Guidelines for the diagnosis and management of pericardial diseases: The Task Force for the Diagnosis and Management of Pericardial Diseases of the European Society of Cardiology

(ESC) Endorsed by: The European Association for Cardio-Thoracic Surgery (EACTS). Eur Heart J. 2015;36:2921–64.
8. Fabre A, Sheppard MN. Sudden adult death syndrome and other nonischaemic causes of sudden cardiac death. Heart. 2006;92:316–20.
9. Childs H, Friedrich MG. Cardiovascular magnetic resonance imaging in myocarditis. Prog Cardiovasc Dis. 2011;54(3):266–75.
10. Friedrich MG, Marcotte F. Cardiac magnetic resonance assessment of myocarditis. Circ Cardiovasc Imaging. 2013;6(5):833–9.
11. Sinagra G, Anzini M, Pereira NL, Bussani R, Finocchiaro G, Bartunek J, Merlo M. Myocarditis in clinical practice. Mayo Clin Proc. 2016;91(9):1256–66.
12. Biesbroek PS, Hirsch A, Zweerink A, van de Ven PM, Beek AM, Groenink M, Windhausen F, Planken RN, van Rossum AC, Nijveldt R. Additional diagnostic value of CMR to the European Society of Cardiology (ESC) position statement criteria in a large clinical population of patients with suspected myocarditis. Eur Heart J Cardiovasc Imaging. 2017; https://doi.org/10.1093/ehjci/jex308.
13. Ferreira VM, Piechnik SK, Dall'Armellina E, Karamitsos TD, Francis JM, Choudhury RP, Friedrich MG, Robson MD, Neubauer S. Non-contrast T1-mapping detects acute myocardial edema with high diagnostic accuracy: a comparison to T2-weighted cardiovascular magnetic resonance. J Cardiovasc Magn Reson. 2012;14:42.
14. Ferreira VM, Piechnik SK, Dall'Armellina E, Karamitsos TD, Francis JM, Ntusi N, Holloway C, Choudhury RP, Kardos A, Robson MD, Friedrich MG, Neubauer S. Native T1-mapping detects the location, extent and patterns of acute myocarditis without the need for gadolinium contrast agents. J Cardiovasc Magn Reson. 2014;16:36.
15. Huber AT, Bravetti M, Lamy J, Bacoyannis T, Roux C, de Cesare A, Rigolet A, Benveniste O, Allenbach Y, Kerneis M, Cluzel P, Kachenoura N, Redheuil A. Non-invasive differentiation of idiopathic inflammatory myopathy with cardiac involvement from acute viral myocarditis using cardiovascular magnetic resonance imaging T1 and T2 mapping. J Cardiovasc Magn Reson. 2018;20(1):11.
16. Friedrich MG, Sechtem U, Schulz-Menger J, et al. Cardiovascular magnetic resonance in myocarditis: a JACC White Paper. J Am Coll Cardiol. 2009;53:1475–87.
17. Imazio M. Pericarditis with troponin elevation: is it true pericarditis and a reason for concern? J Cardiovasc Med (Hagerstown). 2014;15:73–7.
18. Imazio M, Brucato A, Spodick DH, Adler Y. Prognosis of myopericarditis as determined from previously published reports. J Cardiovasc Med (Hagerstown). 2014;15:835–9.
19. Aquaro GD, Perfetti M, Camastra G, Monti L, Dellegrottaglie S, Moro C, Pepe A, Todiere G, Lanzillo C, Scatteia A, Di Roma M, Pontone G, Perazzolo Marra M, Barison A, Di Bella G, Cardiac Magnetic Resonance Working Group of the Italian Society of Cardiology. Cardiac MR with late gadolinium enhancement in acute myocarditis with preserved systolic function: ITAMY study. J Am Coll Cardiol. 2017;70(16):1977–87.
20. Di Bella G, Camastra G, Monti L, Dellegrottaglie S, Piaggi P, Moro C, Pepe A, Lanzillo C, Pontone G, Perazzolo Marra M, Di Roma M, Scatteia A, Aquaro GD. Working group 'Cardiac Magnetic Resonance' of the Italian Society of Cardiology. Left and right ventricular morphology, function and late gadolinium enhancement extent and localization change with different clinical presentation of acute myocarditis Data from the ITAlian multicenter study on MYocarditis (ITAMY). J Cardiovasc Med (Hagerstown). 2017;18(11):881–7.

Cardiac Transplantation

7

Contents

7.1 Introduction and Possible Role of CMR in the Follow-Up of Cardiac Transplantation

Cardiac allograft rejection (CAR) is a major complication in the first year after cardiac transplantation affecting 40% of patients with at least one episode. CAR is responsible of death in 12% and increases the subsequent risk of death up to 4 years and, moreover, is an independent risk factor for cardiac allograft vasculopathy (CAV).

Early detection of CAR is a major challenge in clinical practice. In clinical practice, the currently applied protocols include right ventricular endomyocardial biopsy (EMB) that is considered the gold standard for the early diagnosis of CAR.

Currently EMB is associated with serious complications only in less than 1% of cases using the new flexible bioptomes. In cardiac transplanted patients, EMB is used routinely for immediate and for long-term allograft rejection surveillance and, at the moment, has not been replaced by gene expression profiling or any other non-invasive tests [1].

Echocardiography is a useful tool for monitoring CAR, being easily accessible, bedside, and cost- and time-saving. However, the currently used echocardiographic indices, including left ventricular dimensions/function, wall thickness and mass and pericardial effusion, are insensitive markers of CAR [1].

A joint EACVI/Brazilian cardiovascular imaging writing group committee provided a practical guide to echocardiographers involved in the follow-up of heart transplant patients [2]. A comprehensive echocardiographic study at 6-month

M. Imazio et al., *Learning Cardiac Magnetic Resonance*,
https://doi.org/10.1007/978-3-030-11608-8_7

post-cardiac transplantation as a baseline and quantification of cardiac chamber size, RV systolic function, both systolic and diastolic parameters of LV function and pulmonary artery pressure is recommended, while subsequent echocardiographic studies should be evaluated in comparison with the findings of the 6-month study. An echocardiographic study without any change, compared with the baseline study, has a high negative predictive value for CAR [2].

No single systolic or diastolic parameter can reliably diagnose CAR. However, if some parameters are abnormal, the potential of CAR is higher. Global longitudinal strain (GLS) is a reliable parameter to diagnose subclinical CAR, applied for serial evaluations and can be used in association with EMB to monitor an acute CAR [1, 2].

CMR has several advantages over echocardiography: it is the gold standard for the evaluation of biventricular volumes and function and allows non-invasive tissue characterization (detection of myocardial edema and scar).

T2 relaxation time is the most widely used CMR index to detect CAR grade ≥2. An increase in T2 relaxation time is directly proportional to myocardial water content. Studies in animal transplant models showed a positive correlation between the increase of T2 relaxation time, histological severity of CAR and ex vivo myocardial water content. Finally, T2 relaxation time improvement has been observed after immunosuppressive therapy [1].

According to a meta-analysis study, T2-STIR intensity and T1-early relative myocardial contrast enhancement were used to detect CAR and improve significantly the diagnostic capability on ruling out clinically significant CAR with a higher sensitivity and negative predictive value (NPV) compared with a single parameter test [3].

LGE sequences are commonly used to evaluate myocardial scars. Currently, there are no studies showing a correlation between LGE and CAR. Although in a recent study CMR-derived myocardial scar and right ventricular end-diastolic volume index (RVEDVI) were independently associated with CV outcomes in transplanted patients [4], CMR-derived myocardial scar and RVEDVI are also independently associated with CV outcomes in transplanted patients during 5-year follow-up [5].

A combination of threshold right ventricular end-diastolic volume index and edema values can predict a positive EMB with very good accuracy (sensitivity, 93%; specificity, 78%; positive predictive value, 52%; and negative predictive valve, 98%) [1]. CMR is more sensitive than EMB at predicting clinical rejection (sensitivity of 67% vs. 58%), and therefore it can be used as a screening test, before routine EMB [1]. However, while CMR provided novel insight into the myocardial injury associated with transplantation, it was not able to accurately detect acute CAR, as diagnosed by biopsy during this period [1].

At present there is limited research to support routine use of CMR as screening test before EMB in asymptomatic patients; nevertheless, the field is evolving and the combined use of different CMR techniques (cine, T2w, EGE and LGE, perfusion study) may be helpful in the future to select patients for EMB.

The rapid development of molecular tests and new imaging techniques in both echocardiography and CMR in parallel with the use of high sensitivity troponin may be of value for the selection of transplanted patients, who are candidates for EMB.

According to these principles, in a recent review, a detailed evaluation of biochemical, molecular and imaging indices (including those derived from CMR) was recommended before the final decision for EMB in asymptomatic patients with suspected CAR [1].

References

1. Mavrogeni SI, Athanasopoulos G, Gouziouta A, et al. Cardiac transplantation: towards a new noninvasive approach of cardiac allograft rejection. Expert Rev Cardiovasc Ther. 2017;15(4):307–13.
2. Badano LP, Miglioranza MH, Edvardsen T, et al. European Association of Cardiovascular Imaging/Cardio-vascular Imaging Department of the Brazilian Society of Cardiology recommendations for the use of cardiac imaging to assess and follow patients after heart transplantation. Eur Heart J Cardiovasc Imaging. 2015;16(9):919–48.
3. Lu W, Zheng J, Pan XD, et al. Diagnostic performance of cardiac magnetic resonance for the detection of acute cardiac allograft rejection: a systematic review and meta-analysis. J Thorac Dis. 2015;7(3):252–63.
4. Krieghoff C, Barten MJ, Hildebrand L, et al. Assessment of subclinical acute cellular rejection after heart transplantation: comparison of cardiac magnetic resonance imaging and endomyocardial biopsy. Eur Radiol. 2014;24:2360–71.
5. Butler CR, Kim DH, Chow K, et al. Cardiovascular MRI predicts 5-year adverse clinical outcome in heart transplant recipients. Am J Transplant. 2014;14(9):2055–61.

Pericardial Diseases

8

Contents

8.1 The Normal Pericardium

The **pericardium** (from the Greek περί, "around," and κάρδιον, "heart") is a double-walled sac containing the heart and the roots of the great vessels.

The normal pericardium is composed of two layers: an outer fibrous layer (parietal pericardium) and an inner serous later (visceral pericardium or epicardium) covering a variable content of fibrous and fat tissue and coronary arteries and closely connected to the myocardium (Fig. 8.1) [1].

The reflection of the visceral pericardium into the parietal pericardium over the great vessels is responsible for the creation of spaces, where pericardial fluid can accumulate and they can be seen on imaging. Greater spaces are called **sinuses**, while smaller spaces between adjacent anatomic structures are called **recesses**. The main sinuses include the **transverse sinus**, located between the aorta and

M. Imazio et al., *Learning Cardiac Magnetic Resonance*,
https://doi.org/10.1007/978-3-030-11608-8_8

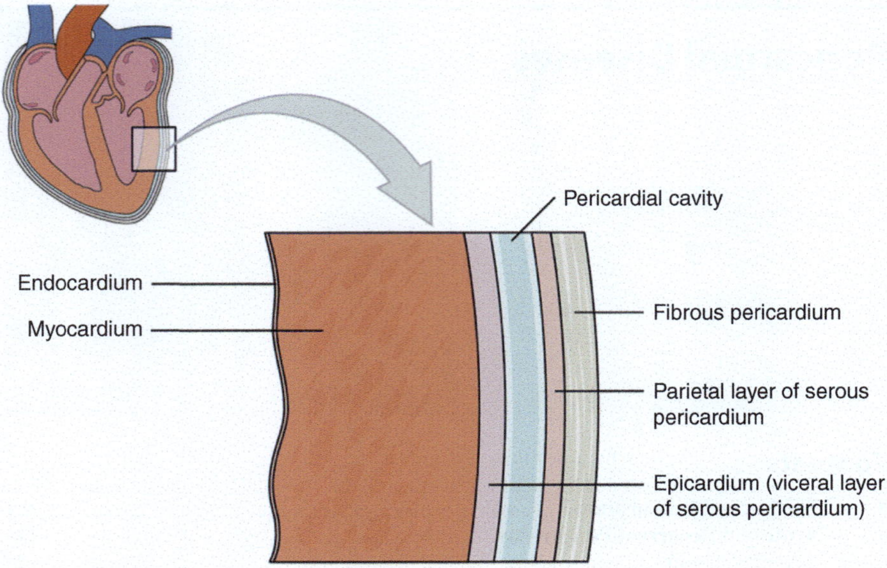

Fig. 8.1 Pericardial layers and cavity (Source: En Wikipedia)

pulmonary trunk anteriorly and the atria and veins posteriorly, and the **oblique sinus** located behind the left atrium and between the pulmonary veins and the inferior vena cava (Fig. 8.2) [1].

In physiological conditions a small amount of fluid (10 to 50 mL) of plasma ultrafiltrate, produced by the visceral pericardium itself, lubricates the two layers allowing continuous movements without attrition. Moreover the pericardium is relatively anelastic and has a modest compressive effect on the heart chambers, thus limiting chamber dilatation (especially for right chambers) and affecting the degree of atrioventricular valve insufficiencies.

Diastolic filling is affected by the pericardium, and such filling is especially affected in pericardial diseases, when either compressive pericardial effusion (cardiac tamponade or moderate to large pericardial effusion or constrictive pericarditis) or rigid pericardium (constriction) may affect diastolic filling and ventricular coupling [1].

On CMR, black-blood T1-weighted spin-echo sequences allow the best approach to visualize the pericardium. The normal pericardium is visible as a thin (<3 mm thick), smooth, low-intensity curvilinear structure surrounded by high-intensity mediastinal and epicardial fat and medium-intensity myocardium (Fig. 8.3, panel a). The pericardium is best seen adjacent to right chambers since the contrast is higher with surrounding fat tissue; on the contrary the low signal of lung parenchyma and the paucity of surrounding fat make difficult the visualization of the pericardium adjacent to left ventricle [2–4].

In b-SSFP cine CMR, the pericardium is seen to have a low signal intensity, while pericardial fluid has a high-intensity signal (Fig. 8.4, panel b).

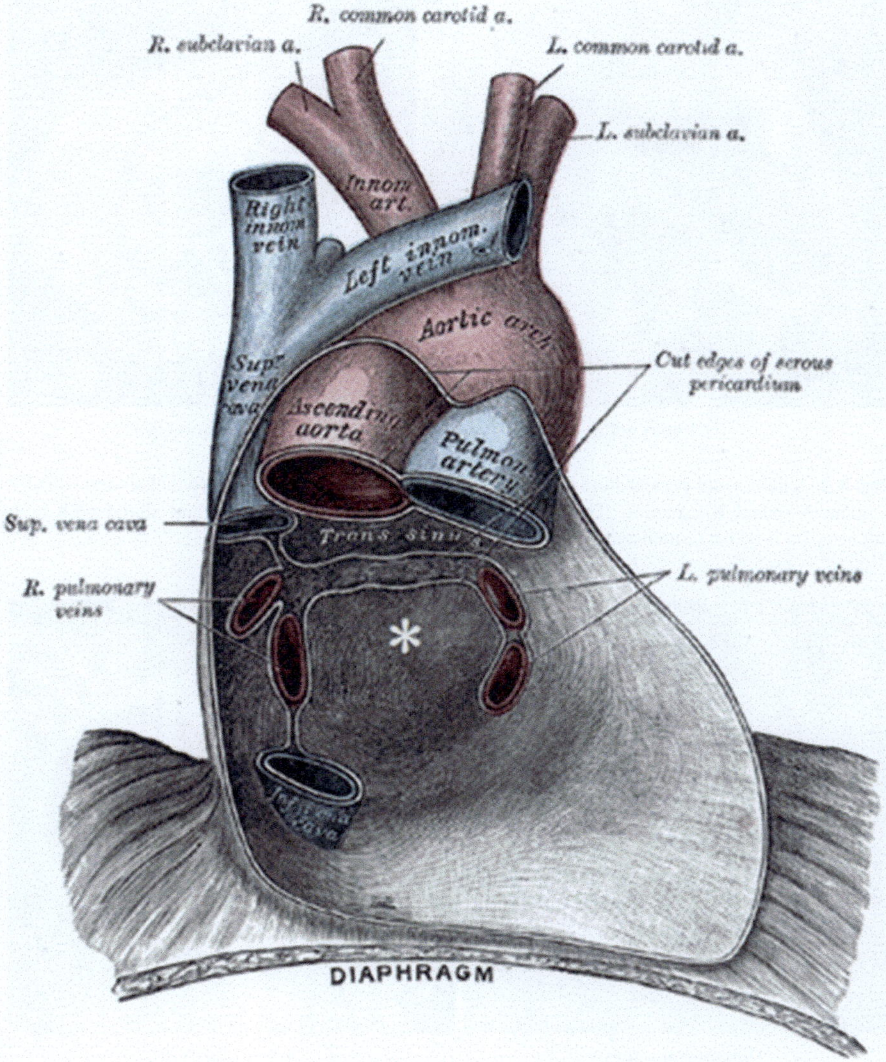

Fig. 8.2 Pericardial sinuses are main pericardial recesses formed by reflections of the pericardium over vascular and cardiac structures. The **transverse sinus** is between the aorta, pulmonary trunk and the atria and pulmonary veins. The oblique sinus (*) is posterior to the left atrium and between the inferior vena cava and pulmonary veins (Source: En Wikipedia)

On CMR, the normal pericardium is about 1.2 mm thick at diastole and 1.7 mm thick at systole, and on this basis the normal pericardium is <3 mm. Overall, it overestimates the real thickness that is up to 1 mm in anatomical studies. This overestimation is explained by pericardial layers motion, lack of spatial resolution and chemical-shift artefacts at the fat-fluid interface. In physiological conditions, no pericardial fluid is detected during the entire cardiac cycle (diastole and systole), but minimal amount can be only seen during systole [2–4].

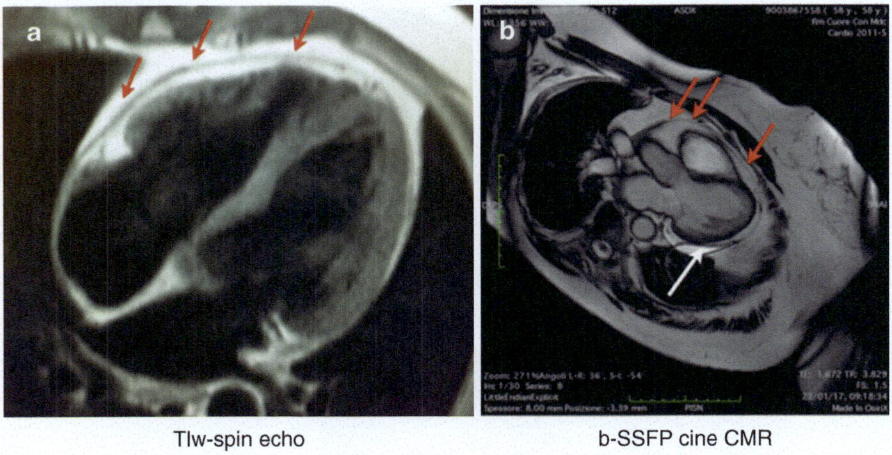

Fig. 8.3 The normal pericardium (red arrows) on T1-weighted spin-echo (panel **a**) and b-SSFP sequences (panel **b**) imaging. The white arrow indicates the pericardial fluid signal with high intensity on b-SSFP sequences (see text for explanation)

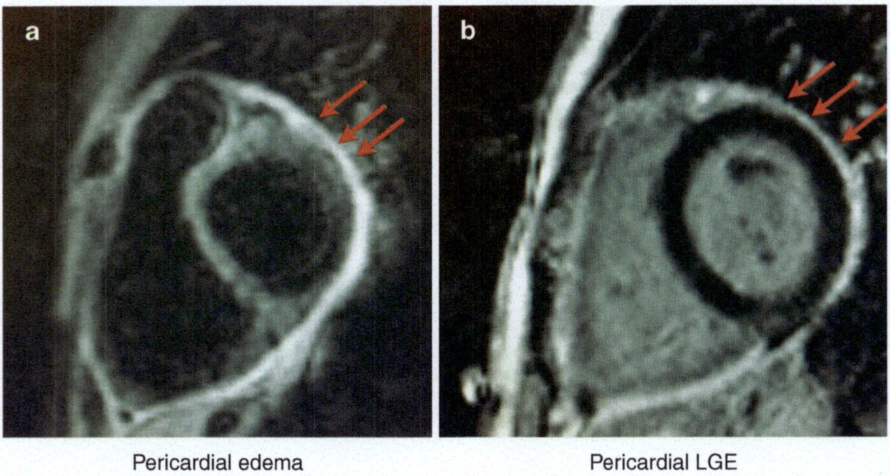

Fig. 8.4 CMR criteria for pericarditis include (1) pericardial thickening, (2) pericardial edema, (3) pericardial effusion and (4) pericardial LGE. In this figure it is depicted pericardial edema on T2w-imaging (panel **a**) and pericardial LGE (see text for additional explanation). Reproduced with permission form Imazio M. Myopericardial Diseases, Springer 2016

8.2 Acute and Recurrent Pericarditis

8.2.1 Acute Pericarditis

The inflamed pericardium is edematous and may be thickened. On this basis, the same features that can be observed in myocarditis for the myocardium can be also detected during pericarditis for the pericardium [4–9].

Current 2015 ESC guidelines on the management of pericardial diseases underline that CMR can be used to confirm the diagnosis in doubtful cases when clinical criteria are not sufficient for the diagnosis [5].

CMR criteria for acute pericarditis (Fig. 8.4) include:

1. Pericardial thickening on T1-weighted spin-echo imaging or cine CMR
2. Pericardial edema on T2-weighted STIR spin-echo imaging (increased signal of the inflamed pericardium)
3. Pericardial effusion
4. Pericardial late gadolinium enhancement (LGE) as evidence of increased vascularization and extracellular space (that may be related to edema in the acute phase or fibrosis in chronic forms) and vascularization

The diagnostic accuracy of such criteria has not been extensively studied.

About 25% of patients with pericarditis may have increased levels of troponins and concomitant myocarditis that can be mild and associated with normal biventricular function and wall motion (myopericarditis) or reduced ventricular function and abnormal wall motion (perimyocarditis). In these cases, CMR can be very helpful to assess the presence of concomitant myocarditis (see chapter on myocarditis) [5]. Tagging CMR techniques may allow to depict fibrotic adhesions of pericardial layers.

8.2.2 Recurrent Pericarditis

In patients with recurrent pericarditis (defined according to the 2015 ESC guidelines criteria as *recurrence of pericarditis after a symptom-free interval of 4 to 6 weeks*) (time for the anti-inflammatory therapy and its tapering) after a previous attack of pericarditis, the same CMR diagnostic criteria of acute pericarditis can be adopted. In the absence of a symptom-free interval of at least 4 to 6 weeks, the term *incessant pericarditis* should be adopted to describe a pericarditis without resolution of symptoms after conventional medical therapy [5].

8.3 Pericardial Effusion and Cardiac Tamponade

CMR can detect the presence or even small amount of pericardial fluid and may allow to attempt the characterization of pericardial fluid on the basis of the appearance of pericardial fluid on T1-weighted, T2-weighted and cine imaging. As a general rule, a transudate has a higher content of water and shows a high signal on cine imaging and T2-weighted still images compared with a low signal on T1-weighted still images, while an exudate has a higher content of proteins and cells and thus has a higher signal on T1-weighted still images compared with cine imaging and T2-weighted images (Table 8.1).

Nevertheless, motion artefacts make pericardial fluid characterization less reliable.

Table 8.1 CMR signal features of pericardial fluid on different sequences (see text for explanation)

	T1w	Cine/T2w
Transudate	Low	High
Exudate	High	Not homogeneous
Haemorrhage	Not homogeneous	Not homogeneous
Chylopericardium	High	High/low

Cardiac tamponade is often a life-threatening condition or potentially so, thus requiring a quick evaluation and triage that cannot be offered by CMR. On this basis, CMR is not indicated for the evaluation of potentially unstable patients, and echocardiography (even at bedside) is the imaging test of choice for such patients [5, 6].

8.4 Constrictive Pericarditis

In constrictive pericarditis the pericardium is thickened (≥3 mm) in about 80% of cases, and CMR is helpful to detect pericardial thickness as well as signs of increased ventricular interdependence on cine real-time imaging (Figs. 8.5 and 8.6) and evidence of pericardial inflammation (high signal on T2w-images and pericardial LGE) that may be reversible with empiric anti-inflammatory therapy in up to 50% of cases [5, 6].

On the contrary CMR is not indicated for the evaluation of pericardial calcifications that are better assessed by CT. The presence of calcifications is not uncommon in the setting of constrictive pericarditis and suggests a long-term and chronic process with indication to pericardiectomy, if possible and indicated.

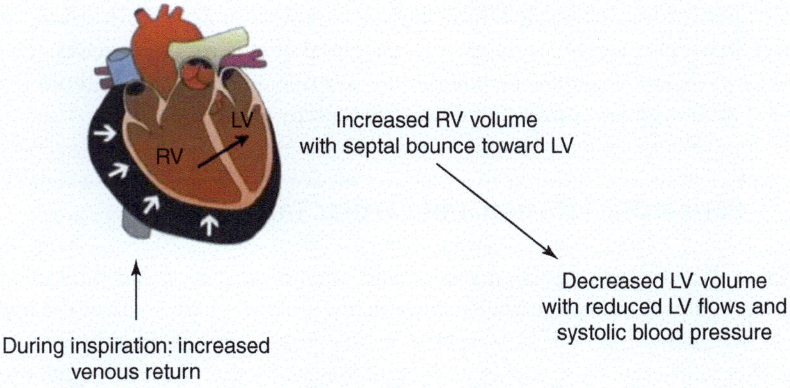

Fig. 8.5 Increased ventricular interdependence in constrictive pericarditis

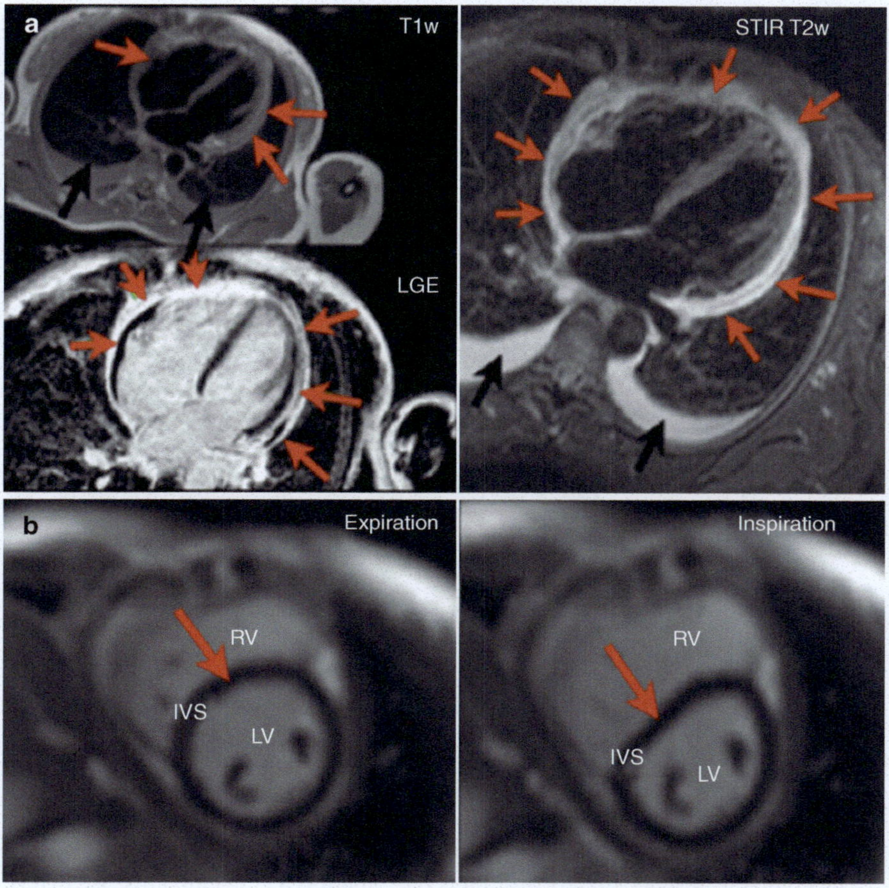

Fig. 8.6 A case of constrictive pericarditis in the setting of acute inflammation of the pericardium as can be demonstrated by CMR. See pericardial thickening on T1w image, pericardial edema on STIR T2w image and pericardial LGE (panel **a**) as well as inspiratory flattening of the interventricular septum as evidence of increased ventricular interdependence on cine real-time images (panel **b**)

8.5 Pericardial Masses and Congenital Diseases

A simple classification of these entities that are not so common in clinical practice is reported in Table 8.2.

Congenital defects of the pericardium usually affect the left section of the heart and may be associated with other congenital abnormalities (e.g. interatrial septal defects, patent ductus arteriosus, bicuspid aortic valve, pulmonary malformations).

Table 8.2 Pericardial masses and congenital diseases of the pericardium

Congenital diseases	Pericardial defects (partial or complete) Congenital cysts and diverticula
Masses	Tumours • Primary (very rare: 50% of cases are represented by pericardial mesothelioma) • Secondary (common: especially lung cancer, breast cancer, lymphoma and leukaemia, melanoma, extension of cancer from contiguous organs) • Cysts • Congenital • Acquired (especially *Echinococcus*) Haematoma

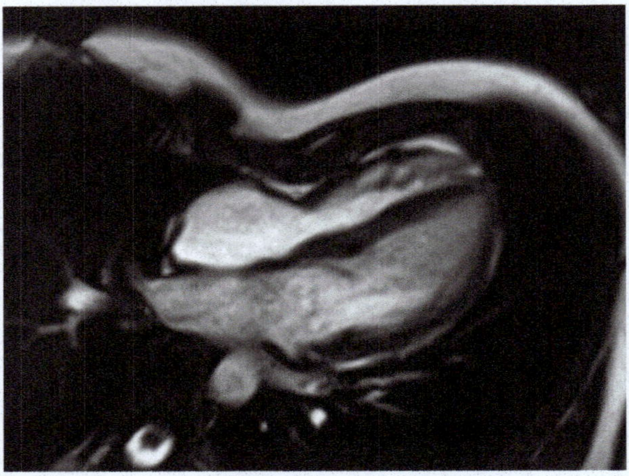

Fig. 8.7 A case of pericardial agenesis: the pericardium cannot be seen as think line with ipointense signal on T1-weighted imaging

The complete absence of pericardium is rare, and it is a congenital disease that is compatible with a normal duration of life. The absence of the pericardium that exerts a constraining effect on cardiac chambers (especially right chambers) is responsible for a dilatation of right chambers with abnormal motility and displacement that may mimic a disease of the right heart (e.g. arrhythmogenic CMP of the RV). ECG is usually altered with RBB and right deviation of the QRS axis. On CMR, the absence of the pericardium can be well assessed on T1w imaging since the usual thin pericardial line within the epicardial fat is not seen (Fig. 8.7).

Partial agenesis of the pericardium is potentially more dangerous since the herniation of cardiac structures through a pericardial defect may be responsible of strangulation and mechanical effect on the herniation with symptoms.

Congenital cysts of the pericardium are defects of the normal development of the pericardium. They are rare (1:1000.000) and more common in the right cardiophrenic angle (50–70% of cases). Pericardial cysts have a round or elliptical shape with variable dimensions from few cm to >20 cm with well-defined contours and without communication with the pericardial cavity. They are usually asymptomatic, an occasional finding on imaging. Possible (rare) complications are infections and haemorrhage with possible increase of size and symptoms related to the compressive effect on surrounding anatomical structures.

On CMR pericardial cysts have a high signal intensity on T2w images and cine imaging (see following case).

Pericardial masses will be discussed in the specific chapter on masses.

8.6 Case 1: Acute Pericarditis

Case presentation: A 40-year-old Caucasian female patient, with unremarkable past medical history, presented to the emergency department with pleuritic chest pain radiating to the trapezius ridge, exacerbated by breathing and relieved by leaning forward; the symptoms were accompanied by fever (up to 38.5 °C). Physical examination was negative, blood pressure was 100/60 mmHg without paradoxical pulse and neither jugular venous distention nor pericardial friction rub was detected. Electrocardiogram (ECG) showed right bundle branch block, minimum ST-segment elevation in aVL lead and negative T waves in anterior leads. Serum C-reactive protein level was elevated, and hs-troponin T levels were not detectable. Chest X-ray showed moderate bilateral pleural effusion and cardiac silhouette in the upper limit of normal range. Echocardiography revealed mild to moderate pericardial effusion, measuring up to 10 mm (largest telediastolic echo-free space). There were no echocardiographic signs of right atrial or right ventricular compression, and mitral flow velocity variation was normal, but the inferior vena cava was dilated (21 mm) and not collapsing. The left ventricular contractile function was normal, and there were no wall motion abnormalities. Acute pericarditis was diagnosed.

Patient was admitted to hospital (one high-risk feature with fever >38 °C), and etiological screening was negative. Symptoms responded very slowly to oral indomethacin and colchicine, fever persisted, with elevated levels of inflammatory indices, and mild signs of visceral congestion developed.

Cardiac magnetic resonance imaging (CMR) was performed in order to better evaluate the pericardium and the myocardium and to exclude the evolution towards constriction.

CMR findings: Cardiac MRI showed severe diffuse pericardial thickening with marked signs of inflammation at T2-weighted short-tau inversion recovery (STIR) images and extensive post-contrast enhancement of the pericardium (Fig. 8.8). No myocardium enhancement was detected. No significant pericardial effusion was found. Dynamic tagging images showed localized pericardial adhesion between inflamed visceral and parietal pericardial surfaces.

Free-breathing, real-time cine images showed inspiratory septal flattening, indicating mild accentuation of interventricular interdependence (Fig. 8.9). CMR also showed bilateral pleural effusion and dilatation of the inferior vena cava with slow flow. Steroid therapy (prednisone 0.5 mg/kg/day) was introduced, with rapid positive clinical response and followed by slow tapering (reducing the daily dose of 2.5 mg every 2 weeks) after remission.

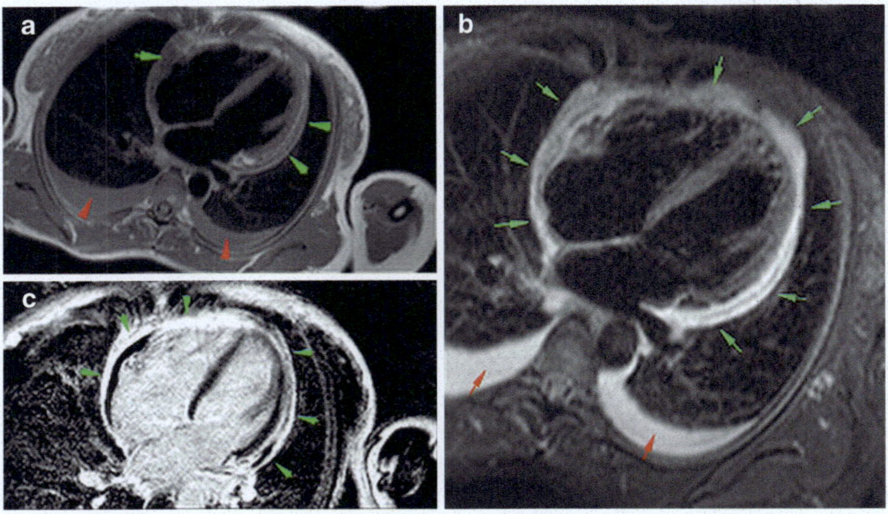

Fig. 8.8 T1-weighted image (panel **a**), four-chamber view, showing thickened pericardium (green arrows) and bilateral pleural effusion (red arrows). STIR T2-weighted image (panel **b**), four-chamber view, showing hyperintense signal of the pericardial layers (green arrows); bilateral pleural effusion (red arrows). Post-contrast image (panel **c**), four-chamber view, showing late enhancement of the pericardium (green arrows)

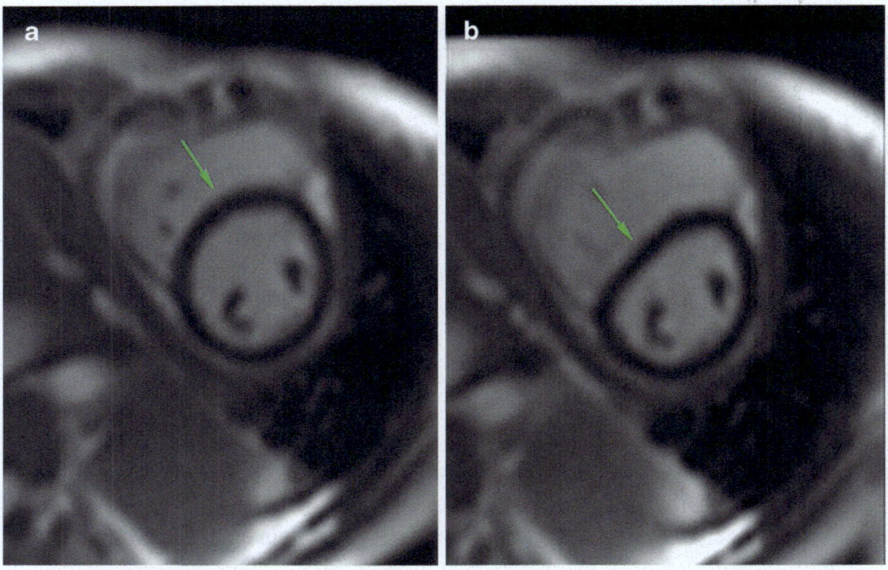

Fig. 8.9 Real-time, free-breathing cine images, mid-ventricular short-axis view, in expiration (panel **a**) and inspiration (panel **b**), showing inspiratory septal flattening (panel **b**), indicating accentuated interventricular interdependence

Conclusions: The final diagnosis was acute idiopathic pericarditis because of the negativity of etiological diagnostic testing.

The patient underwent cardiac MRI in order to exclude the evolution towards a constrictive form and to assess the degree of increased pericardial thickness and functional effects of the pericarditis. Black-blood T1-weighted spin-echo cardiac MRI was used for morphological assessment of the pericardium, the intrathoracic and mediastinal structures. Increased signal intensity of the pericardium on T2W-STIR images confirmed active inflammation. Late gadolinium enhancement of the pericardium is coherent with the acute inflammatory state. Real-time cine images during free-breathing demonstrated the presence of a modest septal bounce, indicating accentuation of interventricular interdependence. This finding is related to reduced distensibility of the inflamed and thickened pericardium and usually disappears with the resolution of the inflammatory process.

8.7 Case 2: Constrictive Pericarditis

Case presentation: A 38-year-old man with a history of a recent incessant pericarditis with direct evolution in constrictive pericarditis with distended jugular veins, ascites and leg edema was referred for CMR to assess pericardial thickness and the presence of pericardial inflammation before pericardiectomy.

CMR findings: The pericardium was thickened on T1-weighted imaging with a maximum value of 4 mm, and there were no signs of pericardial edema on T2-weighted images (no evidence of active inflammation). Mild pericardial LGE was detected as evidence of previous pericarditis with fibrosis (Fig. 8.10).

Conclusions: In the setting of constrictive pericarditis, CMR is useful to evaluate pericardial thickness, signs of ventricular interdependence and pericardial inflammation to prevent early pericardiectomy before complete resolution of pericardial inflammation, a potentially reversible cause of constriction.

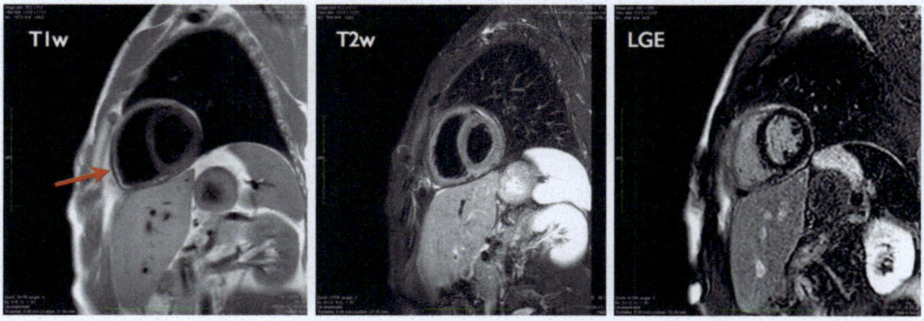

Fig. 8.10 A case of constrictive pericarditis with mild pericardial thickening on T1w imaging (see red arrow), no pericardial edema on T2w imaging and evidence of pericardial fibrosis on LGE (pericardial LGE without edema)

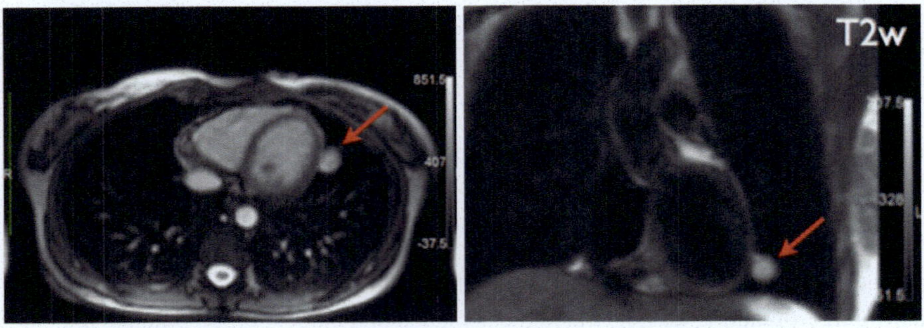

Fig. 8.11 A case of a simple, uncomplicated pericardial cyst with high signal on cine and T2w imaging (see red arrows)

8.8 Case 3: Pericardial Cyst

Case presentation: A 24-year-old woman was referred for CMR with a suspicion of pericardial cyst detected on chest X-ray as incidental finding. The patient was asymptomatic.

CMR findings: On CMR, the pericardial cyst was evident on cine imaging with a typical high signal on T2w imaging reflecting the watery content (Fig. 8.11).

Conclusions: An uncomplicated cyst is a round structure with well-defined borders and high content of water if uncomplicated. On this basis an uncomplicated pericardial cyst has a high signal on cine and T2w imaging.

8.9 Key Points and CMR Protocol

- The normal pericardium can be hardly seen as a low-intensity line within the epicardial fat on T1-weighted imaging with a thickness of <3 mm.
- T1-weighted imaging allows to study pericardial thickness that is increased if >3 mm.
- T2-weighted imaging detects pericardial edema as a bright signal from the pericardium.
- The normal pericardium is not highly vascularized, and in the presence of chronic inflammation and fibrosis, the extracellular space of the pericardium is increased with neovascularization producing pericardial LGE.
- Due to motion artefacts, CMR is not able to fully characterize the nature of pericardial fluid. Transudate have high signal on cine and T2w imaging but low signal on T1w imaging, while exudates have a higher content of proteins and cells with dishomogeneous signal on T1w and low signal on T2w imaging.
- In case of constrictive pericarditis, CMR allows the assessment of pericardial thickness, inflammation and signs of increased ventricular interdependence (septal bounce).
- A complete protocol for the evaluation of the pericardium includes cine sequences, cine real time, T1w and T2w imaging as well as LGE (Table 8.3).

Table 8.3 Standard protocol for the evaluation of the pericardium

Sequence	Data
Cine	Evaluation of kinesis and septal bounce as well as presence of pericardial and pleural effusion
TSE T1 weighted	Anatomical assessment of the pericardium and its thickness (normal if less than 3 mm)
STIR T2 weighted	Evaluation of the presence of possible pericardial and myocardial edema
LGE	Assessment of active pericardial inflammation (if associated with edema) or chronic inflammation and fibrosis (pericardial LGE only)
Cine real time	Evaluation of increased ventricular interdependence in constrictive pericarditis
Perfusion	Evaluation of perfusion of a pericardial mass (if sign of malignancy is present)

References

1. Misselt AJ, Harris SR, Glockner J, Feng D, Syed IS, Araoz PA. MR imaging of the pericardium. Magn Reson Imaging Clin N Am. 2008;16(2):185–99.
2. Bogaert J, Francone M. Cardiovascular magnetic resonance in pericardial diseases. J Cardiovasc Magn Reson. 2009;11:14.
3. Imazio M. Myopericardial diseases. Springer; 2016.
4. Imazio M, Pedrotti P, Quattrocchi G, Roghi A, Badano L, Faletti R, Bogaert J, Gaita F. Multimodality imaging of pericardial diseases. J Cardiovasc Med (Hagerstown). 2016;17(11):774–82.
5. Adler Y, Charron P, Imazio M, et al. European Society of Cardiology (ESC). 2015 ESC Guidelines for the diagnosis and management of pericardial diseases: The Task Force for the Diagnosis and Management of Pericardial Diseases of the European Society of Cardiology (ESC) Endorsed by: The European Association for Cardio-Thoracic Surgery (EACTS). Eur Heart J. 2015;36(42):2921–64.
6. Klein AL, Abbara S, Agler DA, Appleton CP, Asher CR, Hoit B, Hung J, Garcia MJ, Kronzon I, Oh JK, Rodriguez ER, Schaff HV, Schoenhagen P, Tan CD, White RD. American Society of Echocardiography clinical recommendations for multimodality cardiovascular imaging of patients with pericardial disease: endorsed by the Society for Cardiovascular Magnetic Resonance and Society of Cardiovascular Computed Tomography. J Am Soc Echocardiogr. 2013;26(9):965–1012. e15.
7. Bogaert J, Cruz I, Voigt JU, Sinnaeve P, Imazio M. Value of pericardial effusion as imaging biomarker in acute pericarditis, do we need to focus on more appropriate ones? Int J Cardiol. 2015;191:284–5.
8. Imazio M, Gaita F, LeWinter M. Evaluation and treatment of pericarditis: a systematic review. JAMA. 2015;314(14):1498–506.
9. Alraies MC, AlJaroudi W, Yarmohammadi H, Yingchoncharoen T, Schuster A, Senapati A, Tariq M, Kwon D, Griffin BP, Klein AL. Usefulness of cardiac magnetic resonance-guided management in patients with recurrent pericarditis. Am J Cardiol. 2015;115(4):542–7.

Heart Valve Diseases

9

Contents

9.1 CMR Advantages and Limitations in the Study of Heart Valve Diseases

Echocardiography remains the gold standard and first level choice for the study of heart valve diseases because of its availability, high temporal resolution for the study of valvular flows, limited costs and possibility to perform the examination in any condition.

Nevertheless CMR has specific advantages to be considered in specific settings. CMR is the gold standard for the evaluation of biventricular volumes and function, right chamber evaluation and non-invasive tissue characterization for the evaluation of edema and scars [1].

In the study of heart valve diseases, most morphological data are acquired by cine imaging (SSFP), which allows a good contrast between the endocardium, myocardium and blood, the study of the outflow and inflow tracts without any specific limitation also in patient with poor echocardiographic windows. On CMR the evaluation of the planimetry and anatomic area of semilunar valves is easier and more reliable than in echocardiography. The main limitation of CMR remains the limited capability to study flows compared with Echo-Doppler and small mobile masses (e.g. heart valve vegetations and small highly mobile tumours such as papillary

M. Imazio et al., *Learning Cardiac Magnetic Resonance*,
https://doi.org/10.1007/978-3-030-11608-8_9

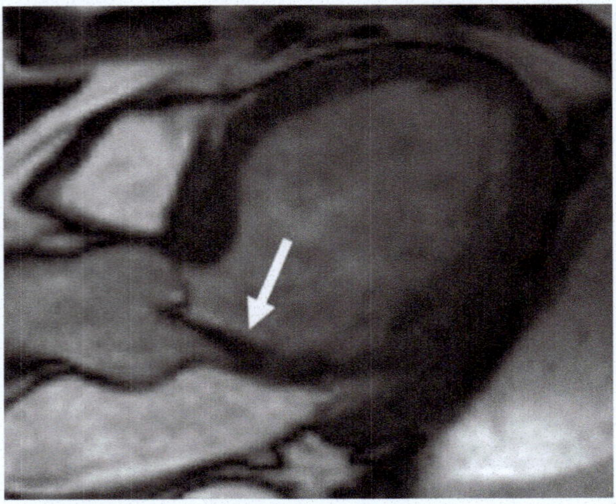

Fig. 9.1 A case of mild aortic regurgitation visualized by cine SSFP in a LVOT section. The regurgitant jet is visualized as a hypointense signal marked by the white arrow. From Myerson Journal of Cardiovascular Magnetic Resonance 2012, 14:7. Open access

Table 9.1 Comparison of CMR vs. echocardiography in the study of heart valve diseases

Study	Echocardiography	CMR
Volumes and function	+++	++++
Myocardial scar	+/−	++++
Concomitant aortic disease	+	++++
Regurgitant jets	+++	+
Quantification of aortic/pulmonary regurgitation	++	+++
Quantification of mitral/tricuspid regurgitation	+++	+
Anatomical area (stenosis)	+	+++
Quantification of valvular stenosis	+++	++
RV heart valve diseases	++	++++

Semiquantitative evaluation: − insufficient, +/− scarce, + sufficient, ++ discrete, +++ good, ++++ very good

fibroelastoma) since temporal resolution of CMR is lower than in echocardiography and CMR sections are 5–8 mm thick that may be too thick for the study of small lesions and valvular structures that are typically 1–2 mm thick. Turbulent flows cannot be correctly visualized on CMR since the loss of phase by protons is visualized as a loss of signal in cine sequences as SSFP (Fig. 9.1). Such jets are more related to accelerations rather than velocities and may be responsible of an underestimation of the valvular disease. On this basis CMR allows more the identification of a mild or severe defect rather than moderate. Gradient sequences are more suitable for the evaluation of the presence and entity of a valvular jet. A summary of the diagnostic capabilities of CMR compared with echocardiography is reported in Table 9.1.

In CMR heart valve disease quantification is made possible by phase contrast sequences. The principle of phase contrast sequences is that moving protons have a phase shift proportional to their velocity compared with other protons. If the velocity of a flow is combined with its section area, it is possible to measure the flow as in Echocardiography. Flow measures are reported in a flow/time graph as illustrated in Fig. 9.2. However, the temporal resolution of CMR is only 25–45 ms and thus inferior to Echo-Doppler [1, 2]. Another important difference with Echo-Doppler is that flow measures are performed with alignment of the ultrasound beams in echocardiography, while in CMR the measure is performed with a cross section of the flow (see also Fig. 9.3). In-plane sequences are performed parallel to the flow in order to identify flows, while the assessment is made through plane perpendicular to

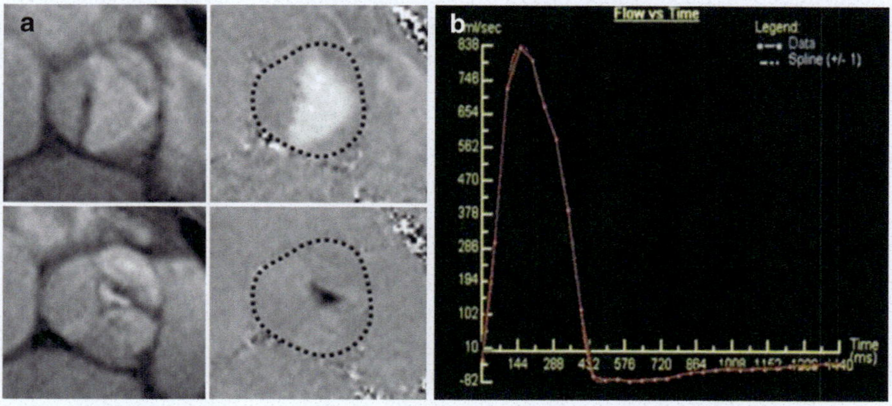

Fig. 9.2 A case of evaluation for aortic flow with mild aortic regurgitation by phase contrast imaging. In panel **a**, anatomic and phase contrast images (the forward aortic flow is white and positive on the graph, while the smaller regurgitant flow is black on the phase contrast image and negative on the flow vs. time curve); in panel **b** flow vs. time curve. The ratio between the backward flow and the forward flow is a direct measure of the regurgitant ratio. From Myerson Journal of Cardiovascular Magnetic Resonance 2012, 14:7. Open access

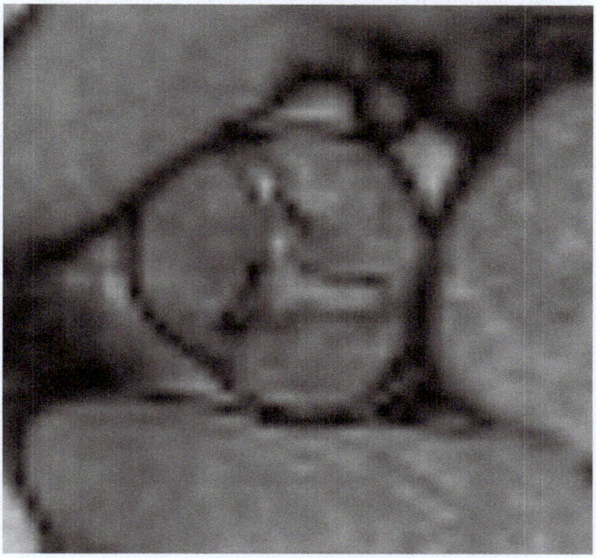

Fig. 9.3 An example of planimetric assessment of the morphology of the aortic valve (tricuspid valve in this case), where it is also possible to evaluate the planimetric area (anatomic valve area) for the quantification of aortic stenosis. From Myerson Journal of Cardiovascular Magnetic Resonance 2012, 14:7. Open access

Table 9.2 Comparison of Echo-Doppler vs. CMR in the study of heart valve diseases

	Echo-Doppler	Phase contrast (CMR)
Temporal resolution	High (about 2 ms)	Low (>20–25 ms)
Capability to assess velocity	High	Low (especially if >3.5 m/s)
How flow is studied	Parallela al flusso	Ortogonale al flusso
Acquisition time	Fast	Slow

the jet direction. Echo-Doppler has a higher temporal resolution (few ms) and a better capability to assess higher velocities, especially if >3.5–4.0 m/s, when CMR measures become less precise because of the loss of signal due to turbulent flow (Table 9.2).

9.2 Left-Side Heart Valve Diseases

Aortic stenosis can be evaluated on CMR especially as anatomic valve area that can be measured by planimetry on a short axis of the valve (Fig. 9.3). Aortic valve velocities >3.5 m/s cannot be evaluated appropriately by CMR. In the study of aortic stenosis, CMR is superior to echocardiography for the anatomic evaluation of the valve (bicuspid vs. tricuspid valve), its planimetry (assessment of anatomic valve area), the evaluation of the aorta, the study of concomitant myocardial scars (detected in about 1/3 of cases at the level of the IV septum), biventricular volumes and function [2, 3].

Aortic regurgitation can be assessed by quantitative analysis identifying the regurgitant jet by in-plane scans, and then the flow is assessed by a through plane phase contrast scan that is conducted perpendicular to the jet (see Fig. 9.4). The regurgitant fraction (RF) can be assessed by the ratio between the backward and forward flow [2].

A regurgitant ratio >33% can identify patients with a significant aortic regurgitation who are prone to develop symptoms and require surgery within few years [4]. Table 9.3 summarizes referral quantitative values for the evaluation of heart valve diseases by CMR. Such values are mainly derived from echocardiography.

Mitral valve diseases can be studied by CMR. Nevertheless the complexity of mitral valve apparatus and lower temporal resolution of CMR, compared with echocardiography, make CMR a second option, and echocardiography is easier to use and allows a complete evaluation and more precise quantification than CMR, if we consider also the possibility of evaluation by transesophageal echocardiography and 3D echo.

Quantification of mitral regurgitation is more precise with echocardiography but can be obtained also by CMR with measure of the regurgitant volume and regurgitant fraction by estimation of LV stroke volume minus forward aortic flow or comparison of LV and RV stroke volumes (see Fig. 9.5) [1, 5, 6].

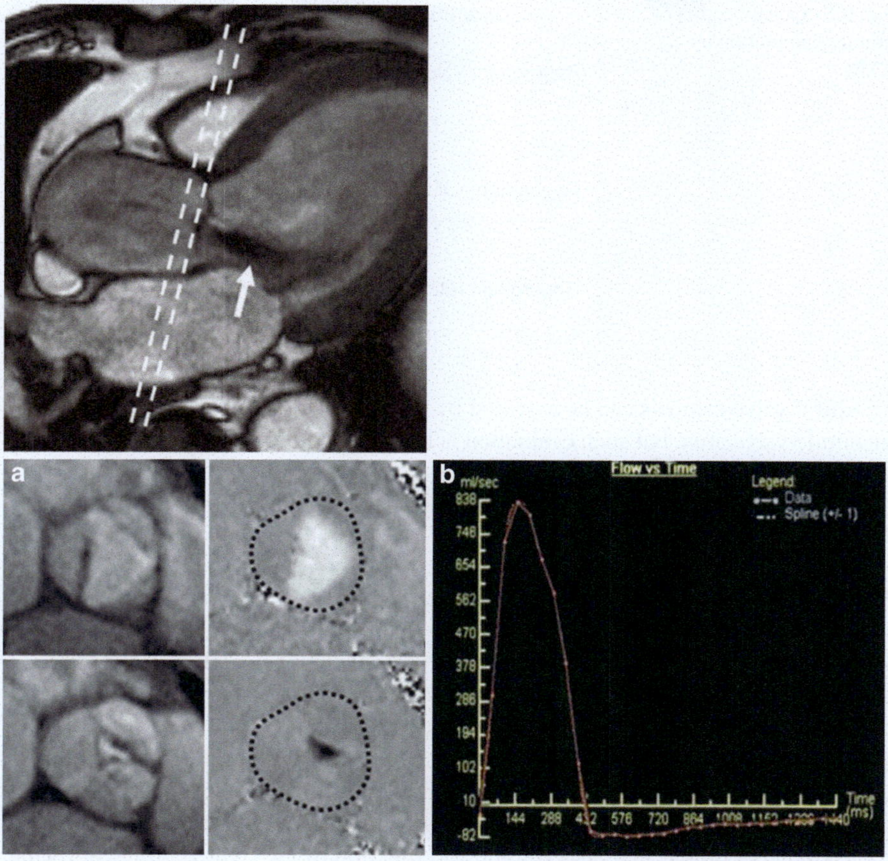

Fig. 9.4 An example of quantitative assessment of an aortic regurgitation: the regurgitant flow is evaluated by a through plane scan, and a flow/time curve is made. The ratio between the regurgitant flow and the forward flow is the regurgitant ratio. From Myerson Journal of Cardiovascular Magnetic Resonance 2012, 14:7. Open access

Table 9.3 Referral quantitative values for the evaluation of heart valve diseases by CMR [5]

Heart valve diseases	Parameter	Mild	Moderate	Severe
Aortic and pulmonary stenosis	Peak velocity (m/s)	<3	3–4	>4
	Anatomical area (cm^2)	>1.5	1.0–1.5	<1.0
Aortic insufficiency	Regurgitant ratio (%)	<30	30–49	>49
	Regurgitant volume (mL)	<30	30–59	>59
Pulmonary insufficiency	Regurgitant ratio (%)	<25	20–35	>35
	Regurgitant volume (mL)	<30	30–40	>40
Mitral and tricuspid stenosis	Anatomical area (cm^2)	>1.5	1.0–1.5	<1.0
Insufficienza mitralica	Frazione di rigurgito (%)	<30	30–49	>49
	Volume di rigurgito (mL)	<30	30–59	>59

Fig. 9.5 Quantification of mitral regurgitation by CMR

Quantification of mitral valve regurgitation

Regurgitant Volume =

LV Stroke volume - Aortic forward flow

Regurgitant volume =

LV Stroke volume - RV stroke volume

Regurgitant ratio (%) =

(Regurgitant volume/LV Stroke volume) × 100

Mitral valve stenosis can be assessed by planimetry of valve area to measure the anatomic valve area, but such evaluation is less precise than the estimation of aortic valve area (Table 9.3).

A case of evaluation of mitral valve area is depicted in Fig. 9.6.

9.3 Right-Side Heart Valve Diseases

CMR is the gold standard for the evaluation of right chambers volumes and function and allows a good evaluation and quantification of pulmonary valve regurgitation can be better estimated by CMR than echocardiography.

The evaluation and quantification of pulmonary valve regurgitation is similar to that outlined for the aortic valve. In the follow-up of operated patients with Fallot disease, CMR allows to quantify the pulmonary regurgitation (a common sequela of the cardiac operation) and also volume and function of the right ventricle allowing to define the time of subsequent interventions before deterioration of the right ventricle.

A pulmonary regurgitation is severe with a regurgitant ratio >35%, and intervention should be considered before significant dilatation of the RV (RV telediastolic volumes <160 mL/m^2) [7]. A case of pulmonary regurgitation during follow-up of operated Fallot is depicted in Fig. 9.7.

Pulmonary stenosis can be evaluated by CMR establishing the anatomical level (subvalvular, valvular and supravalvular), and quantification is performed by planimetry of the valve area as for aortic stenosis.

Tricuspid valve regurgitation can be quantified by evaluation of the regurgitant volume and fraction as outlined for mitral valve (Fig. 9.8).

9.4 Key Points and Protocols

- In the study of heart valve diseases, CMR offers specific advantages: better accuracy in the evaluation of biventricular volumes and function, possibility of tissue characterization (scar assessment) and more accurate quantification of aortic and pulmonary regurgitation than echocardiography.

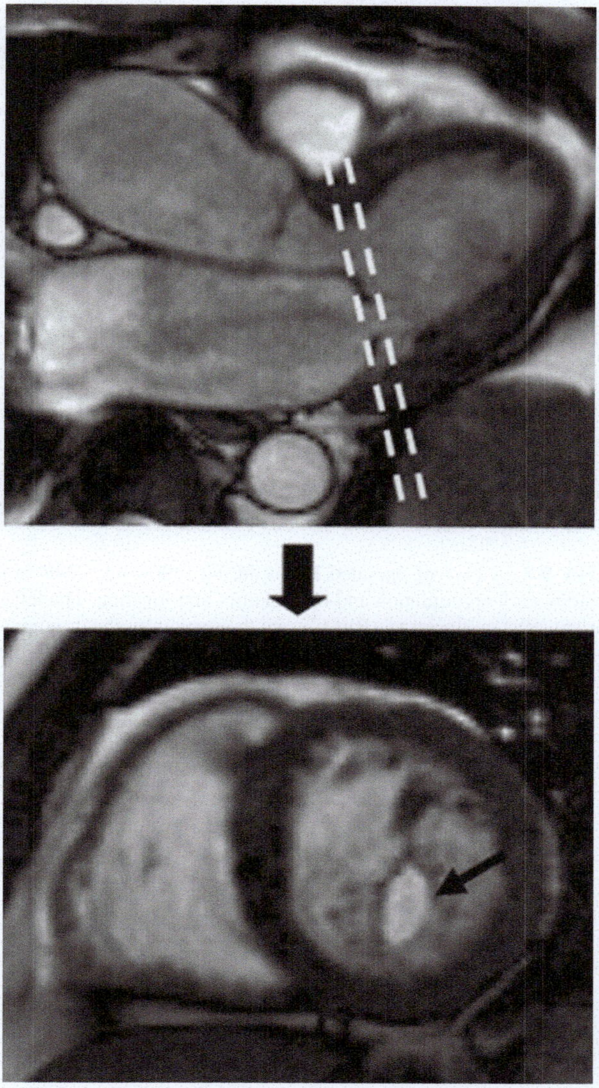

Fig. 9.6 A patient with mitral stenosis: valve area (see black arrow) is obtained and can be measured by planimetry from cine images. From Myerson Journal of Cardiovascular Magnetic Resonance 2012, 14:7. Open access

- Specific limitations of CMR in this setting are represented by lower temporal resolution than echocardiography (Doppler) and inaccurate estimation of high flow velocities making the evaluation of stenosis less precise.
- The initial evaluation of heart valve diseases starts with cine sequences (cine SSFP) for the evaluation of valvular jets. Then quantification of flows is possible by phase contrast sequences that allow to estimate velocities of flows and flows by estimation of the section area of jets (jet flow = jet velocity × jet area).
- The anatomic assessment of semilunar valve morphology is accurate by CMR as with transesophageal echocardiography.
- Aortic and pulmonary stenosis are especially evaluated as planimetry of the valvular area.

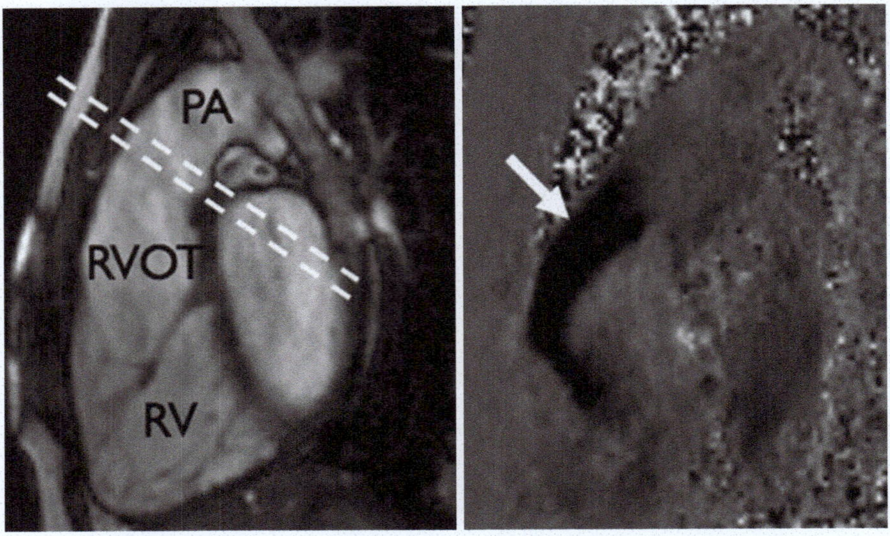

Fig. 9.7 A case of operated Fallot during follow-up. CMR is performed for the evaluation of pulmonary regurgitation and RV volumes and function. The left panel shows a cine image of the right (RV) outflow tract (RVOT), and the section for the through plane section by the use of phase contrast sequences is shown in white lines. On the right panel, the white arrow shows the hypointense signal from severe pulmonary regurgitation. From Myerson Journal of Cardiovascular Magnetic Resonance 2012, 14:7. Open access

Fig. 9.8 Quantification of tricuspid regurgitation

Quantification of mitral valve regurgitation

Regurgitant volume =

RV Stroke volume - Forward pulmonary flow

Regurgitant volume =

RV Stroke volume - LV Stroke volume

Regurgitant ratio (%) =

(Regurgitant volume/RV Stroke volume) × 100

- Aortic and pulmonary regurgitations can be evaluated by CMR with direct estimation of the regurgitant volumes and ratio allowing a more precise quantification than echocardiography.
- Due to the complexity of the mitral valve apparatus, mitral valve diseases can be more easily and accurately evaluated by echocardiography considering not only transthoracic but also transesophageal and 3D echocardiography.
- Quantification of mitral valve regurgitation can be performed by the estimation of the regurgitant volume and ratio.
- A standard CMR protocol for the evaluation of a patient with heart valve disease includes cine SSFP and phase contrast sequences.

References

1. Myerson SG. Heart valve disease: investigation by cardiovascular magnetic resonance. J Cardiovasc Magn Reson. 2012;14:7.
2. Nayak KS, Nielsen JF, Bernstein MA, Markl M, D Gatehouse P, M Botnar R, Saloner D, Lorenz C, Wen H, S Hu B, Epstein FH, N Oshinski J, Raman SV. Cardiovascular magnetic resonance phase contrast imaging. J Cardiovasc Magn Reson. 2015;17:71.
3. Garcia J, Marrufo OR, Rodriguez AO, Larose E, Pibarot P, Kadem L. Cardiovascular magnetic resonance evaluation of aortic stenosis severity using single plane measurement of effective orifice area. J Cardiovasc Magn Reson. 2012;14:23.
4. Myerson SG, D'Arcy J, Mohiaddin R, Greenwood JP, Karamitsos TD, Francis JM, Banning AP, Christiansen JP, Neubauer S. Aortic regurgitation quantification with cardiovascular magnetic resonance predicts clinical outcome. Heart. 2011;97:A93–4.
5. Kawel-Boehm N, Maceira A, Valsangiacomo-Buechel ER, Vogel-Claussen J, Turkbey EB, Williams R, Plein S, Tee M, Eng J, Bluemke DA. Normal values for cardiovascular magnetic resonance in adults and children. J Cardiovasc Magn Reson. 2015;17:29.
6. D'Arcy J, Christiansen JP, Mohiaddin R, Karamitsos TD, Francis JM, Neubauer S, Myerson SG. Prediction of clinical outcome in asymptomatic mitral regurgitation using CMR. Paris: European Society of Cardiology Congress; 2011.
7. Rebergen SA, Chin JG, Ottenkamp J, van der Wall EE, de Roos A. Pulmonary regurgitation in the late postoperative follow-up of tetralogy of Fallot. Volumetric quantitation by nuclear magnetic resonance velocity mapping. Circulation. 1993;88:2257–66.

Masses and Tumours

10

Contents

10.1 Introduction and CMR Advantages in the Study of Masses and Tumours

Echocardiography remains the first imaging modality for the study of masses, but CMR offers specific advantages that make this exam essential for the evaluation of such diseases [1–3]. Specific advantages of CMR over echocardiography include:

1. Greater field of view than echocardiography (extends to the mediastinum and thorax)
2. Possibility to perform multiple scans without the limitations of echocardiographic windows
3. Higher spatial resolution than echocardiography
4. Possibility of tissue characterization with specific sequences (e.g. fat by T1-weighted imaging, edema by T2-weighted imaging, scar by LGE)
5. Possibility to study perfusion and scars by gadolinium-based contrast agents

It is important to underline that the final etiologic diagnosis of a mass is made by histology, but CMR allows to reach a presumptive diagnostic hypothesis and suggests the possible benign or malignant nature of the mass.

Cardiac tumours are rare (prevalence <0.3% in autoptic series) and usually benign (75% of cases; see also Table 10.1), and masses are more common in clinical practice. Cardiac tumours are especially secondary localization (metastases)

M. Imazio et al., *Learning Cardiac Magnetic Resonance*,
https://doi.org/10.1007/978-3-030-11608-8_10

Table 10.1 Relative frequency of primary tumours of the heart

Benign (75%)	Malignant (25%)
Myxoma (30%)	Angiosarcoma (9%)
Lipoma (10%)	Rhabdomyosarcoma (6%)
Fibroelastoma (10%)	Mesothelioma (4%)
Rhabdomyoma (8%)	Fibrosarcoma (3%)
Fibroma (4%)	Lymphoma (2%)
Hemangioma (3%)	
Teratoma (3%)	

of cancer (20–40 times more common than primary tumours of the heart). Nevertheless the concept of benign/malignant is relative, since even a benign tumour may be responsible of serious consequences in the heart (e.g. arrhythmias, embolic events) [1].

10.2 CMR Protocol for the Study of Masses and Tumours

A comprehensive evaluation of a "mass" should include different CMR sequences to better characterize the nature of the finding [1–5]:

1. SSFP cine sequences (weighted on the ratio T2/T1) allow to identify the mass in at least two orthogonal planes and its morphology, size, mobility and functional consequences (e.g. flow obstruction, reduced contractility)
2. T1-weighted imaging with and without fat saturation to assess the presence of fat
3. T2-weighted imaging to assess the presence of edema and watery content
4. First-pass perfusion after injection of gadolinium-based contrast (0.05–0.1 mmol/kg) to assess if the mass is perfused
5. Early (EGE) and late gadolinium enhancement (LGE) to identify thrombi (as minus within cardiac chambers after injection of contrast), mass perfusion and scars or fibrous tissue

A systematic approach for the evaluation of the mass includes the comparison of at least two orthogonal sections of the mass with the outlined different CMR sequences to attempt a characterization of the "mass" (see Table 10.2). As a general consideration, fat has a high signal on T1-weighted imaging that can be suppressed with "fat suppression" sequences. Neoplastic cells are generally bigger in size and with an increased watery content than normal cells. A neoplastic mass has some degree of edema, inflammation and neovascularization that can be demonstrated on CMR sequences.

Cardiac masses often have more common localizations that may be helpful for the diagnostic evaluation: for instance, the pericardium is a common localization for metastases (see Fig. 10.1).

Although CMR is generally better than echocardiography for the characterization of masses, an important exception is represented by small, highly

Table 10.2 Signal intensity of more common masses on different CMR sequences (comparison with normal myocardium)

Massa cardiaca	T1-weighted[a]	T2-weighted	LGE
Pseudotumour			
Thrombus	Low[b]	Low[b]	No uptake
Pericardial cyst	Low	High	No uptake
Benign			
Myxoma	Isointense	High	Heterogeneous
Lipoma	High[a]	High	No uptake
Fibroma	Isointense	Low	High
Rhabdomyoma	Isointense	Isointense/high	No or minimal
Malignant			
Angiosarcoma	Heterogeneous	Heterogeneous	Heterogeneous
Rhabdomyosarcoma	Isointense	High	Hyperintense
Undifferentiated sarcoma	Isointense	Isointense	Heterogeneous
Lymphoma	Isointense	Isointense	No or minimal
Metastasis[c]	Low	Hyperintense	Heterogeneous

[a]In T1-weighted imaging, fat signal can be suppressed with specific sequences
[b]Thrombus may show high signal if recent
[c]The exception is melanoma that shows a high signal in T1w imaging and low signal on T2w imaging because of high cellularity with low degree of edema

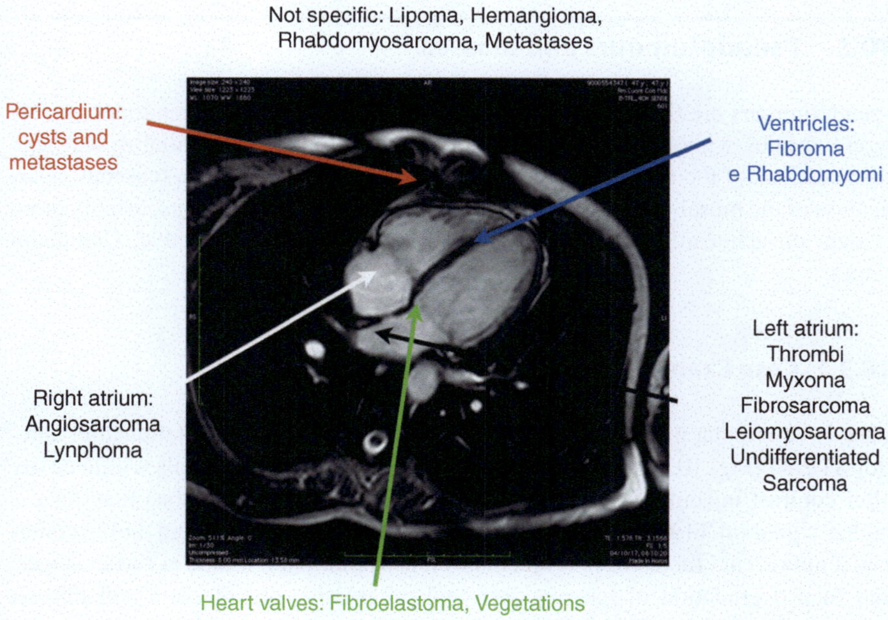

Fig. 10.1 Typical localization of specific masses in cardiac chambers

mobile masses (e.g. valvular vegetations and valvular fibroelastoma). Due to the small size and lower temporal resolution of CMR, echocardiography (especially transesophageal echocardiography) is better than CMR for the study of such masses.

Table 10.3 More common features of a malignant mass

Mass features • Large, especially if >5 cm • Irregular borders • Local invasion • Right chamber localization • Pericardial and/or pleural involvement (e.g. effusion, masses) • Multiple lesions
CMR tissue characterization • Heterogeneous on T1w, T2w imaging (suggests haemorrhage and necrosis) • Haemorrhagic pericardial effusion (high signal on T1w imaging) • Contrast uptake • High signal on T1w imaging and low signal on T2w imaging suggests a metastatic melanoma

Specific features of masses may increase the suspicion of the malignant nature of the mass. A malignant mass is generally bigger (>5 cm) with irregular borders, local invasion and neovascularization and perfused, and it can be associated with pericardial and/or pleural effusions (Table 10.3).

10.3 Pseudotumours and Masses

Pseudotumours are the most common findings in clinical practice and include different entities without a neoplastic significance: thrombi, pericardial cysts, huge calcifications of the mitral annulus especially posterior localization (caseous calcification of the mitral valve), normal variants or development remnants, usually more evident on echocardiography (e.g. Chiari network, Eustachian valve, Coumadin ridge).

10.3.1 Case Examples

Case 1. Ventricular thrombus. A 65-year-old man with a late presentation after anterior STEMI (Fig. 10.2). Thrombi can be seen as low-intensity signals within cavity after contrast injection (EGE and LGE imaging). A recent thrombus may have a higher signal on T1w and T2w imaging, and the signal is attenuated and becomes low if not recent (Table 10.4). A recent thrombus is similar to blood at earlier stages, and then degradation of haemoglobin and progressive organization and fibrosis attenuate the signal on T1w/T2w imaging.

Case 2. A young woman referred to CMR for the evaluation of a pericardial mass. On CMR a pericardial cyst is evident (see short-axis scan with red arrow on the left panel of Fig. 10.3) with typical high intensity of signal on T2w imaging due to watery content in an uncomplicated cyst.

Case 3. A 44-year-old woman evaluated for a mass on echocardiography. On CMR (Fig. 10.4), the mass is located in the left atrium with well-defined borders,

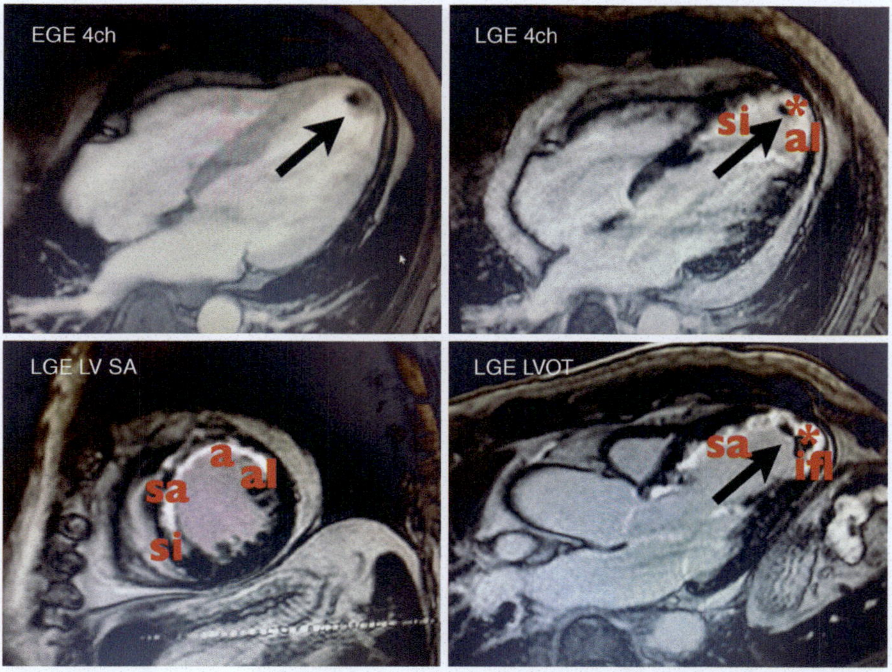

Fig. 10.2 A LV apical thrombus is evident as minus in four chambers scan on EGE and LGE imaging (see black arrow) in the setting of a large myocardial infarction involving the apex, anterior wall and septum (see high signal and evidence of ischemic scar on LGE imaging)

Table 10.4 Evolving CMR features of signal from a thrombus according to time

Thrombus	T1w	T2w	EGE/LGE
Acute	High	High	No uptake
Subacute	High	Low	No uptake
Chronic	Low	Low	No uptake

high signal on T1w/T2w imaging, heterogeneous aspect on cine imaging and LGE suggestive for cardiac myxoma (see also Table 10.2). This is also an example of a benign mass.

Case 4. A 40-year-old man with a known lymphoma and an echocardiographic referral for a ventricular mass infiltrating the left ventricle wall. On CMR (Fig. 10.5), the mass is not well defined within the anterior wall of the LV on cine SSFP, with a high signal on T2w imaging and heterogeneous contrast uptake on LGE imaging suggestive for a secondary localization that was demonstrated to be a secondary myocardial localization of the lymphoma. This is an example of malignant mass.

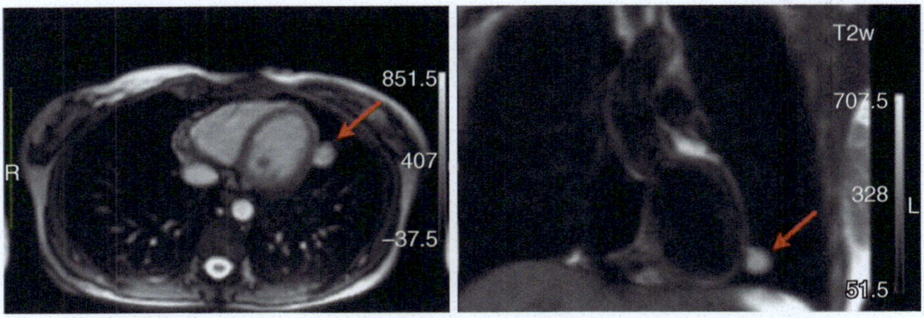

Fig. 10.3 A pericardial cyst (see red arrow on image) with typical high signal on T2w imaging (right panel)

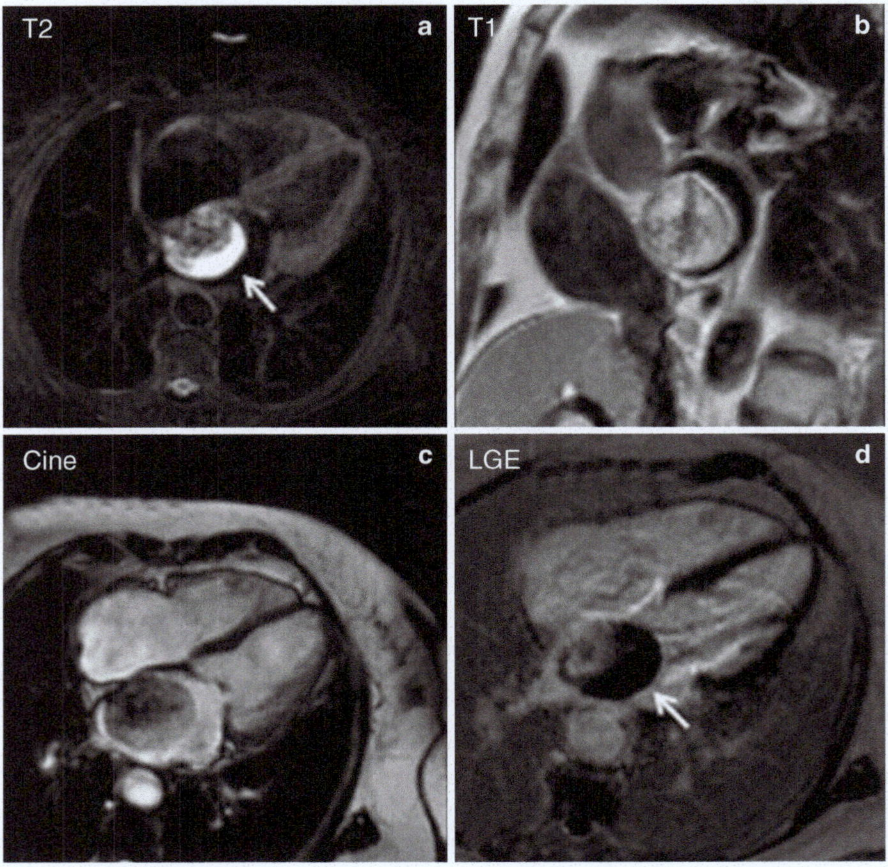

Fig. 10.4 Evaluation of a well-defined left atrial mass with high signal on T1w and especially T2w imaging (suggesting high watery content). Heterogeneous aspect on cine and LGE imaging typical of atrial myxoma

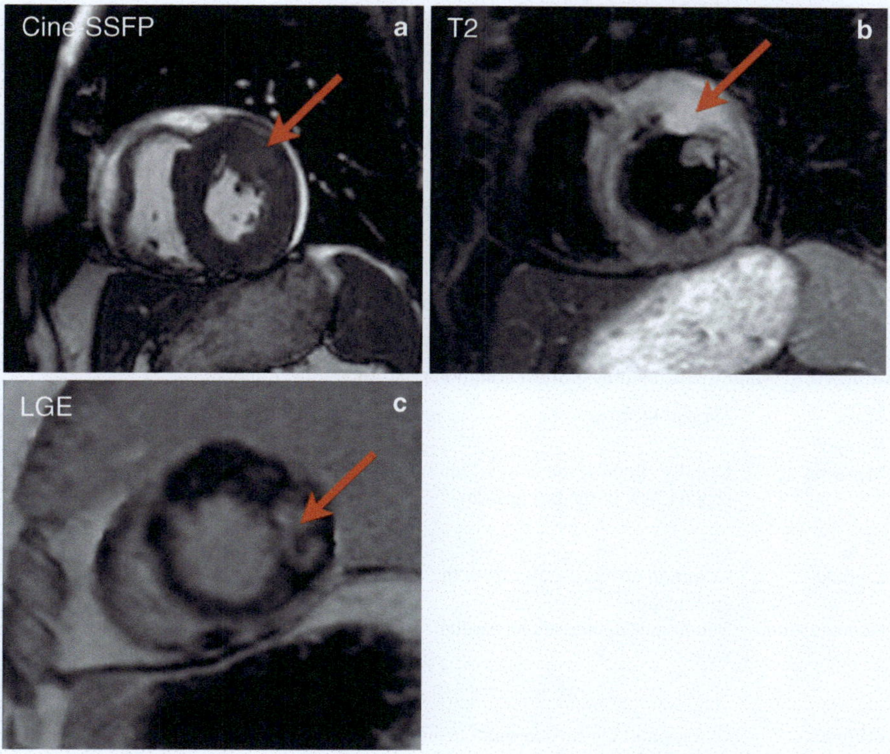

Fig. 10.5 Example of secondary localization of cancer with CMR tissue characterization: infiltrative mass within the anterior wall of the LV (see red arrows) with high signal intensity on T2w imaging and heterogeneous uptake after contrast injection on LGE imaging

10.4 Key Points and Protocols

- In clinical practice the most common masses are thrombi that can be demonstrated as filling defect after contrast injection (on EGE and LGE imaging).
- Cardiac tumours are rare and usually benign (75% of cases: the most common tumour as well as most common benign tumour is atrial myxoma, while the most common primary malignant cardiac tumour is sarcoma); secondary localizations of cancer are most common than primary tumours in clinical practice.
- CMR is superior to echocardiography for the tissue characterization of a mass allowing to offer a better morphological evaluation of the mass (morphology, size, borders, infiltration, tissue characterization, perfusion and contrast uptake).
- Small, highly mobile masses such as valvular vegetations and valvular fibroelastoma are exceptions, since echocardiography is superior to CMR for the study of this subgroup of masses due to its better temporal resolution than CMR.

- CMR features suggestive for a malignant mass include size >5 cm, irregular borders, infiltration, neovascularization and association with pericardial and/or pleural effusions.
- Specific localization may suggest an increased probability of a subset of masses (e.g. metastases more commonly affect the pericardium; see also Fig. 10.1).
- Although CMR is helpful to arise a suspicion of a specific etiology of a mass (Table 10.5), the final diagnosis is always made by histology.
- A standard protocol for the evaluation of a mass includes cine imaging, T1w (with and without fat suppression) and T2w imaging, first-pass perfusion (optional, may be considered) and EGE and LGE imaging (Table 10.6).

Table 10.5 Main CMR features of most common types of cardiac tumours

Mass	Typical localization	CMR signal features
Benign		
Myxoma	Usually single at the level of interatrial septal (75% in the left atrium)	Isointense/high in T1w, high on T2w (water) and heterogeneous after contrast (cystic, haemorrhage, fibrosis, calcifications)
Lipoma	Common (10%) usually from the epicardium	High signal on T1w, no uptake of contrast (low vascularization)
Fibroelastoma	Small, mobile masses on cardiac valves	Better for an echo; on CMR isointense on T1w and high signal on T2w (if seen, may be missed on CMR)
Fibroma	Common in the myocardium, usually as single lesion	Low vascularization: isointense on T1w and low signal on T2w (low watery content), late high signal after contrast
Rhabdomyoma	Common in children, usually within the myocardium with multiple lesions	Isointense (T1w) and high signal on T2w (difference from fibroma)
Hemangioma	High vascularization	High and heterogeneous signal on T1w and T2w and after contrast injection
Sarcoma	More common malignant tumour Usually rhabdomyosarcoma in paediatric age with multiple lesions, in the adult setting angiosarcoma is more common (prevalent involvement of the right atrium)	Rhabdomyosarcoma is isointense on T1w and high and heterogeneous signal on T2w and after contrast Angiosarcoma has high and heterogeneous signal on T1w and T2w and after contrast injection

Table 10.6 Standard CMR protocol for the evaluation of a mass

Sequence	Data
Cine	First assessment of a mass (localization, morphology, size, borders, infiltration, mobility)
T1w with and without fat suppression	Identification of fat, fibrous tissue or CMR features similar to the myocardium
STIR T2w	Evaluation of edema and watery content
EGE	Evaluation of masses within chambers (e.g. thrombi)
LGE	Evaluation of perfusion, scar, fibrous tissue and thrombi

References

1. Motwani M, Kidambi A, Herzog BA, Uddin A, Greenwood JP, Plein S. MR imaging of cardiac tumors and masses: a review of methods and clinical applications. Radiology. 2013;268(1):26–43.
2. Dawson D, Mohiaddin R. Assessment of pericardial diseases and cardiac masses with cardiovascular magnetic resonance. Prog Cardiovasc Dis. 2011;54(3):305–19.
3. Braggion-Santos MF, Koenigkam-Santos M, Teixeira SR, Volpe GJ, Trad HS, Schmidt A. Magnetic resonance imaging evaluation of cardiac masses. Arq Bras Cardiol. 2013;101(3):263–72.
4. Abbas A, Garfath-Cox KA, Brown IW, Shambrook JS, Peebles CR, Harden SP. Cardiac MR assessment of cardiac myxomas. Br J Radiol. 2015;88(1045):20140599.
5. Herzog B, Greenwood J, Plein S, Garg P, Haaf P, Onciul S. Cardiovascular magnetic resonance pocket guide. Disponibile al sito web. https://www.escardio.org/Sub-specialty-communities/European-Association-of-Cardiovascular-Imaging-(EACVI)/Research-and-Publications/CMR-Pocket-Guides.

Adult Congenital Heart Diseases

11

Contents

11.1 Introduction and CMR Advantages in the Study of Congenital Diseases in Grown-Up

CMR has now replaced cardiac catheterization for the study of congenital heart diseases providing both morphological and functional informations [1–5]. In the last 20 years, the use of CMR for the study of congenital heart diseases is greatly increased, providing complementary and adjunctive data to echocardiography and reducing the need for ionizing radiation (CT, cardiac catheterization).

The study of congenital heart diseases is one of the most complex topics, since it requires anatomical, physiological and surgical knowledge (Table 11.1), and it is now a subspecialty also for CMR. A detailed description of each congenital disease is beyond the purpose of the present book. We will review specific advantages of CMR in the study of these conditions, the sequential approach and CMR protocols with some examples from clinical cases.

Compared with echocardiography, CMR offers the opportunity of unrestricted morphological study of congenital diseases by multiple planes of section not limited to echocardiographic windows; moreover CMR is the gold standard for the evaluation of biventricular volumes and function and allows to quantify shunts and attempt non-invasive tissue characterization (Table 11.2) [4].

M. Imazio et al., *Learning Cardiac Magnetic Resonance*,
https://doi.org/10.1007/978-3-030-11608-8_11

Table 11.1 Main surgical operation for congenital heart diseases

Surgical operation	CMR protocol
Blalock-Taussig procedure: surgical procedure used to increase pulmonary blood flow for palliation in duct-dependent cyanotic heart defects like pulmonary atresia, which are common causes of blue baby syndrome. In modern surgery, this procedure is temporarily used to direct blood flow to the lungs and relieve cyanosis while the infant is waiting for corrective or palliative surgery (Fig. 11.1)	Possible complications include stenosis or dilatation of the shunt, PA dilatation and pulmonary hypertension CMR study of Qp/Qs, shunt dimension, flows
Arterial switch: an open-heart surgical procedure used to correct dextro-transposition of the great arteries (**d-TGA**); its development was pioneered by Canadian cardiac surgeon William Mustard, and it was named for Brazilian cardiac surgeon Adib Jatene, who was the first to use it successfully. It was the first method of d-TGA repair to be attempted but the last to be put into regular use because of technological limitations at the time of its conception. The use of the arterial switch is historically preceded by two atrial switch methods: the Senning and Mustard procedures The position of the aorta and pulmonary artery is switched with anterior placement of the pulmonary trunk and reimplantation of the coronaries	Possible complications include obstruction of outflow tracts, pulmonary stenosis, dilatation of the aorta and aortic and pulmonary regurgitations. Coronary stenosis and RV dysfunction. CMR study of biventricular function, aorta and pulmonary artery and aortic and pulmonary regurgitations. Coronary artery study
Rastelli procedure: open-heart surgical procedure developed by Italian surgeon Rastelli at the Mayo Clinic. Indicated for d-TGA, VSD and RV outflow tract obstruction A tunnel is created to direct flow from the LV to the aorta and creating a valvolated conduct from the RV to pulmonary artery	Possible complications: stenosis of conduits, LVOT and residual shunts CMR study to assess patency of conduits, LVOT and RVOT, pulmonary artery and coronary arteries
Mustard/Senning procedure: palliative surgery operation to treat transposition of the great arteries. A baffle – or conduit – is created within the atria that reroutes the deoxygenated blood coming from the inferior and superior vena cava to the mitral valve and therefore to the pulmonary circulation	Possible complications include sinus node dysfunction, atrial arrhythmias, ventricular arrhythmias including sudden cardiac arrhythmic death, heart failure due to anatomically right ventricular failure or venous obstruction at the level of the baffle or caval anatomy CMR study of baffles, RV function and evaluation of tricuspid regurgitation
Fontan procedure: palliative surgical procedure used in children with univentricular hearts (Fig. 11.2). Fontan procedure was performed in patients with tricuspid atresia for the first time in 1968. It involves diverting the venous blood from the inferior vena cava and superior vena cava to pulmonary arteries without passing from the morphologic RV Currently *Glenn procedure* is utilized connecting the superior vena cava to the right pulmonary artery and inferior vena cava to pulmonary artery by a conduit	Possible complications include arrhythmias, thrombosis, pulmonary and systemic embolism and RV dysfunction CMR study of conduits and biventricular function

Table 11.2 A comparison of diagnostic capabilities: echocardiography vs. CMR

Feature	Echocardiography	CMR
Section plans for morphology	Limited to echocardiographic windows	Unlimited
LV volumes and function	++	+++
RV volumes and function	+	+++
Right chambers study	++	+++
Evaluation of flows/shunts	++	+++
Study of scars	0	+++

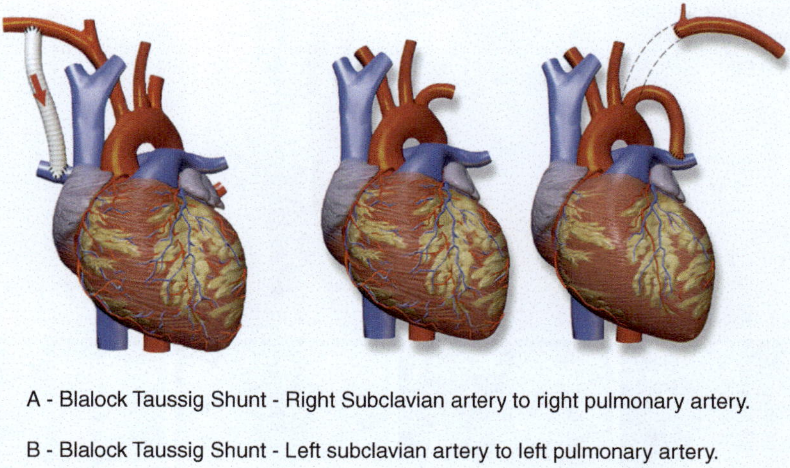

Fig. 11.1 Blalock-Taussig shunt

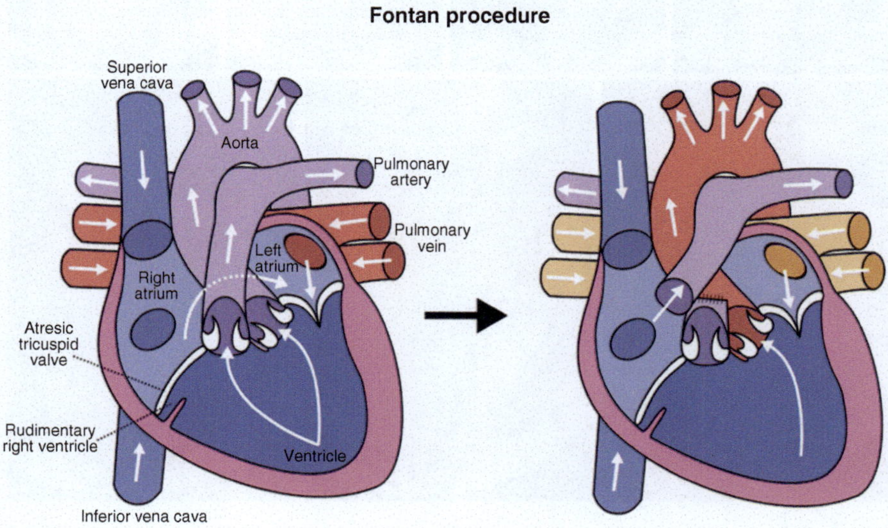

Fig. 11.2 Fontan procedure

Advanced methods by CMR [6] may allow the reconstruction of models of congenital heart diseases by 3D printing (Fig. 11.3). New CMR techniques with 4D flow (Fig. 11.4) may allow to better visualize flows and shunts [7]

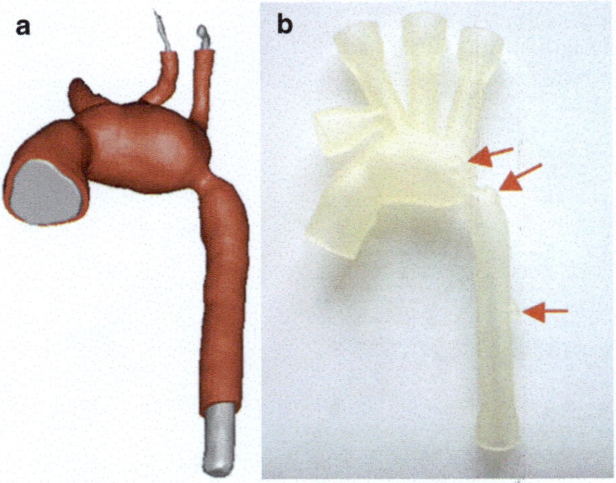

Fig. 11.3 Model of ipoplastic aortic arch from 3D printing from elaboration of CMR imaging. From Biglino et al. Journal of Cardiovascular Magnetic Resonance 2013, 15:2 Open access

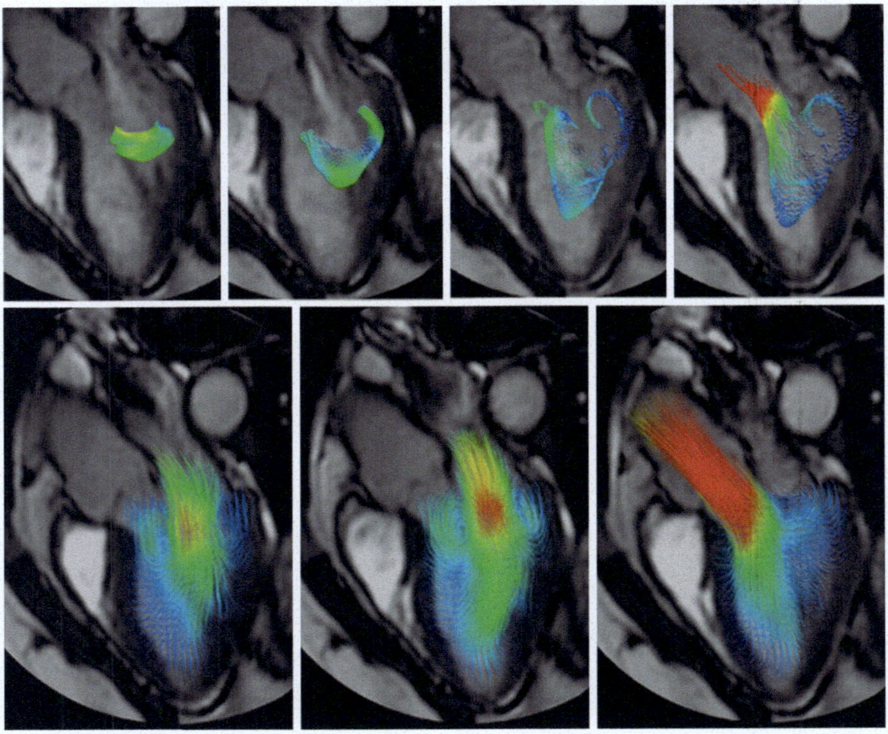

Fig. 11.4 4D flow imaging of intracardiac flows. From Dyverfeldt et al. Journal of Cardiovascular Magnetic Resonance (2015) 17:72. Open access [7]

11.2 Sequential Segmental Approach and CMR for the Study of Congenital Heart Diseases in Adults

CMR allows a more comprehensive morphological study of congenital heart diseases with multiple and unlimited scans from initial conventional planes (sagittal, coronal and axial) according to the specific region of interest and without the limitation of echocardiographic windows. The basic views follow standard scans of the ventricles (see Fig. 11.5).

Starting from long axes, it is possible to acquire short-axis views of both ventricles to assess volume and biventricular function (Fig. 11.6).

By the use of phase contrast sequences, it is possible to calculate forward flow through the aorta (Qs) and pulmonary artery (Qp) in order to assess the Qp/Qs ratio. The same technique can be used also to calculate flows in other sections according to the congenital disease.

The peculiarity of the study of congenital heart disease is the sequential segmental analysis (Fig. 11.7) [8, 9] that consists in a sequential description of the situs (see Fig. 11.8; solitus, inversus, ambiguus), cardiac position (Fig. 11.9; levocardia, dextrocardia, mesocardia), cardiac segments (Fig. 11.10; atria, ventricles, arteries from ventricles) and their connections (Fig. 11.11).

11.3 Main Congenital Heart Disease and Case Examples

The main congenital heart diseases are reported in Table 11.3.

In adults, most common CHDs that can be encountered in clinical practice are:

1. Atrial septal defects
2. Bicuspid aortic valve
3. Corrected tetralogy of Fallot

Case 1. Atrial septal defect. Atrial septal defects are communications between the two atria in the atrial septum, that are usually located at the level of fossa ovalis ["ostium secundum" or fossa-ovalis-type atrial septal defect (ASD)] or just over the AV orifices ("ostium primum" ASD) in the setting of AV septal defects (partial AV canal). The so-called sinus venous defects involving the superior/inferior vena cava or the coronary sinus are rare.

The essential CMR protocol for the study of ASD includes morphological evaluation of cine imaging of 4C, 2C, LVOT, RVOT, SA, atrial SA, phase contrast sequences for aortic and pulmonary arteries to assess the ratio Qp/Qs for the

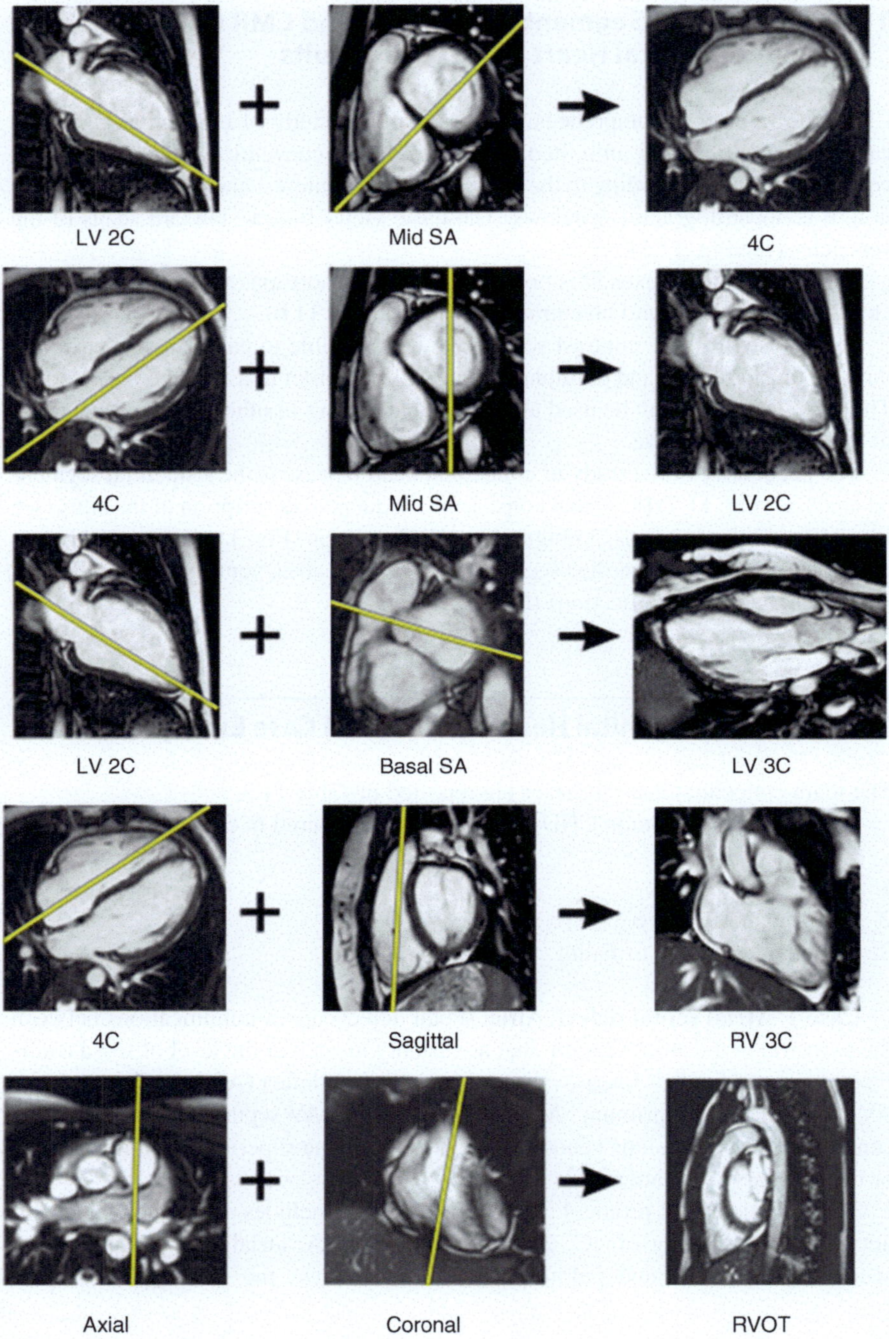

Fig. 11.5 Standard planes for the study of ventricles. 2C, two chambers; 4C, four chambers; 3C, three chambers; RVOT, right ventricle outflow tract. From Fratz et al. Journal of Cardiovascular Magnetic Resonance 2013, 15:51

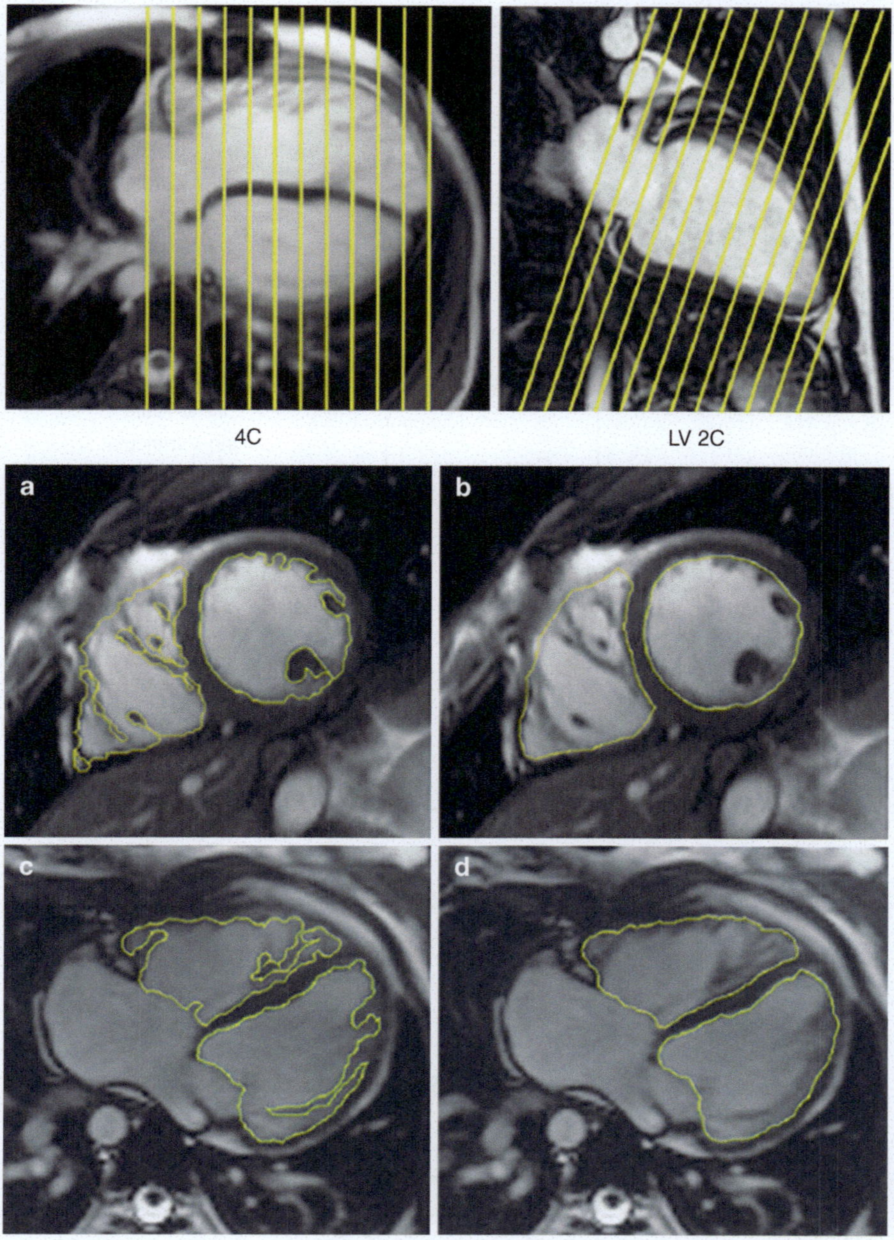

Fig. 11.6 Assessment of short-axis views of the ventricles to calculate volumes and biventricular function

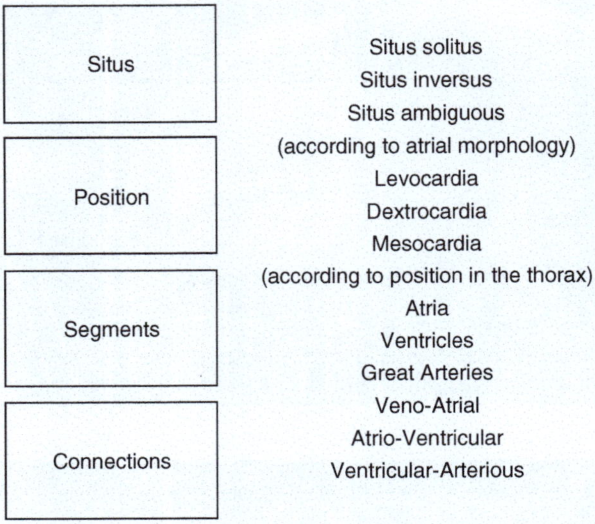

Fig. 11.7 Overview of the sequential segmental analysis for the study of congenital heart diseases. The normal heart can be divided into three segments: atria, ventricles and great arteries, connected to each other at atrioventricular and ventriculo-arterial junctions

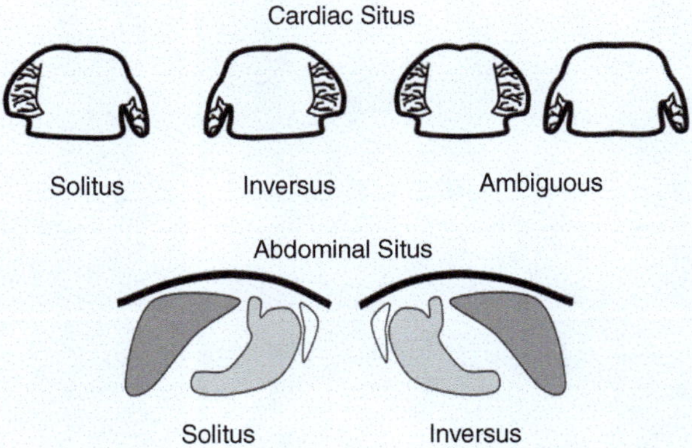

Fig. 11.8 Assessment of cardiac situs (solitus if the right atrium with a right appendage with a broad base is on the right site, while the left atrium with a narrow, tubular appendage is on the left side) and abdominal situs (solitus if the liver is on the right side and the spleen is on the left side)

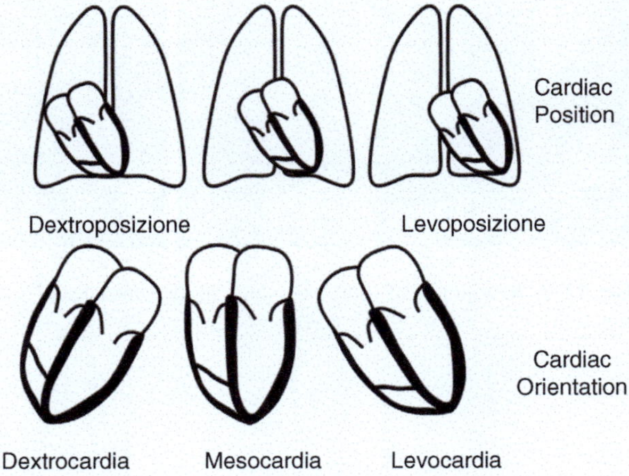

Fig. 11.9 Cardiac position and orientation

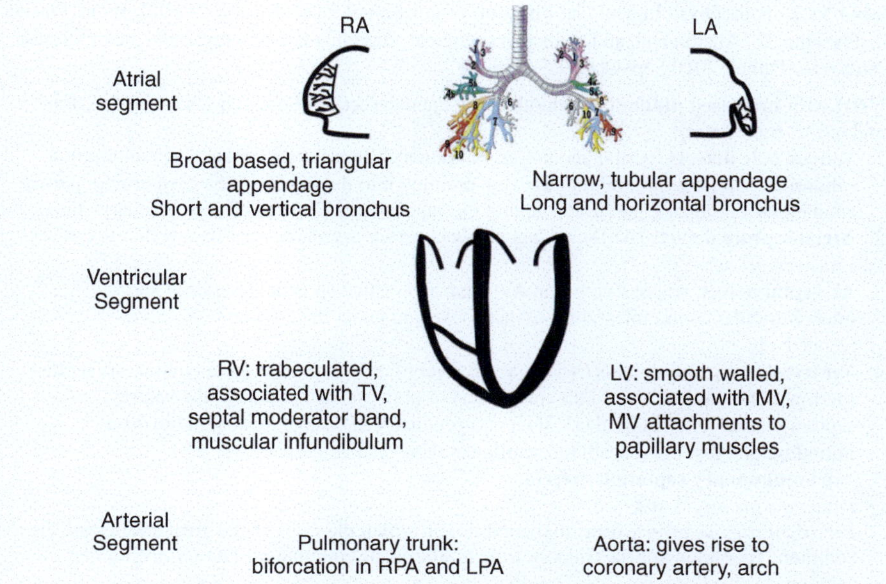

Fig. 11.10 Cardiac segments. *RA* right atrium, *LA* left atrium, *RV* right ventricle, *TV* tricuspid valve, *LV* left ventricle, *MV* mitral valve

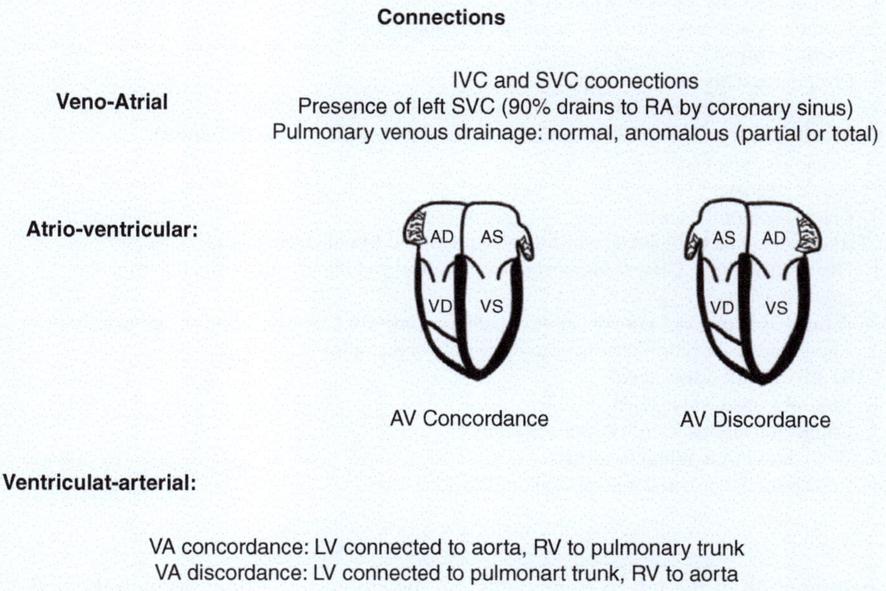

Fig. 11.11 Cardiac connections

Table 11.3 Pathophysiological classification of congenital heart diseases (CHD). From Thiene G, Frescura C. Anatomical and pathophysiological classification of congenital heart disease. Cardiovasc Pathol. 2010 Sep–Oct;19(5):259–74

CHD with increased pulmonary blood flow (septal defects without pulmonary obstruction and left-to-right shunt):
1. **Venous pole defects** (partial anomalous pulmonary venous drainage such as "scimitar syndrome" with the right pulmonary vein draining into the inferior vena cava or with partial anomalous pulmonary vein drainage into the superior vena cava district or coronary sinus)
2. **Atrial septum defects** (ASD): *ostium primum, ostium secundum* or fossa-ovalis-type ASD, *sinus venous defects*
3. **AV septal defect**: where a common AV valve and orifice do exist. Interatrial and interventricular communications are just above and under the common AV valve, respectively
4. **Ventricular septum defects** (VSD): at the level of or well around the membranous septum (perimembranous VSD) or in the inlet apical or outlet muscular part of the ventricular septum musculature (muscular VSDs) or a peculiar VSD is that located in the distal infundibulum, just underneath the semilunar valves (subarterial VSD)
5. **Aortopulmonary septation defects**: *Patent ductus arteriosus*, *Persistent truncus arteriosus* is that condition in which the roots of the great arteries are "in common" (common arterial trunk or truncus arteriosus communis). There is a common semilunar valve ("truncal valve") with a large communication under (VSD) and over the common valve. *Aortopulmonary window*
CHD with decreased pulmonary flow (septal defects with pulmonary obstruction and right-to-left shunt):
1. Pulmonary valve stenosis with ASD
2. Pulmonary stenosis with VSD (tetralogy of Fallot)
3. Tricuspid atresia
4. Ebstein anomaly of the tricuspid valve
5. Single (double-inlet) ventricle with pulmonary stenosis
CHD with obstruction to blood progression and no septal defects (no shunt):
1. Pulmonary stenosis
2. Aortic stenosis
3. Coarctation of the aorta
CHD so severe as to be incompatible with postnatal blood circulation:
1. Ductus-dependent CHD (pulmonary atresia, aortic and mitral atresia and interrupted or atretic aortic arch)
2. Parallel systemic and pulmonary circulations (complete transposition of the great arteries)
3. Anomalous connection/obstruction of the pulmonary veins
CHD silent until adult age:
1. Bicuspid aortic valve (BAV)
2. Congenital anomalies of coronary arteries
3. Wolff-Parkinson-White syndrome
4. Congenitally corrected transposition of the great arteries

quantification of the left to right shunt and the study of the flow through the defect (Fig. 11.12).

Case 2. Bicuspid aortic valve (BAV). Although BAV may be associated with other CHDs (see, for instance, coarctation of the aorta with or without VSD), it may be an isolated defect. Malformation consists of two semilunar aortic cusps with

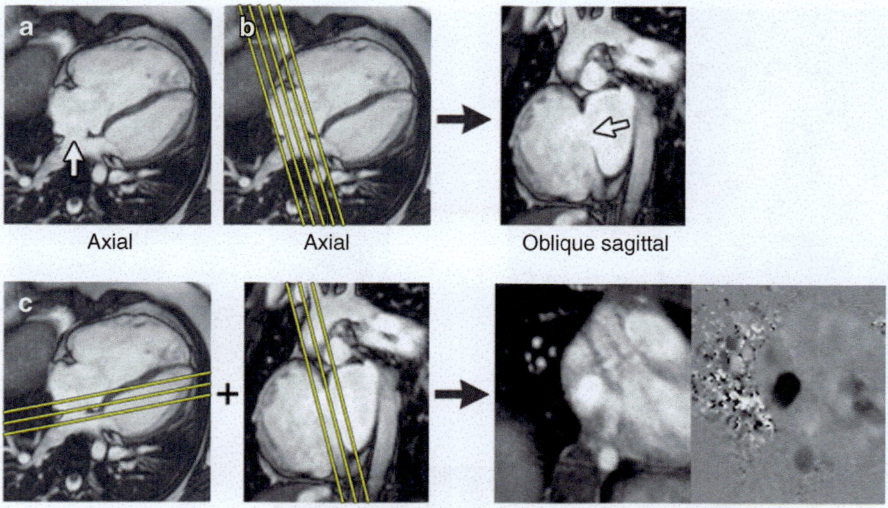

Fig. 11.12 An illustrative case of study of and ASD by CMR (see white arrows). From Fratz et al. Journal of Cardiovascular Magnetic Resonance 2013, 15:51

either side-by-side (laterolateral) or anteroposterior (ventrodorsal) position, which are most probably the result of an embryonic defect of truncal cushions fusion. BAV is frequently associated with dilatation of the ascending aorta and cystic medial necrosis of the tunica media at risk for aortic dissection and sudden unexpected death.

CMR can allow good visualization of the aortic valve morphology by cine imaging from LVOT and LVOT 90° (see Fig. 11.13) also in patients with poor echocardiographic windows and moreover allows the combined study of the aortic root and aorta.

In Fig. 11.14, a CMR imaging of operated coarctation of the aorta is reported.

Case 3. Operated case of tetralogy of Fallot. An embryonic maldevelopment of the truncoconal region determines a malseptation of ventricular outflow at the expense of the pulmonary infundibulum. The infundibular septum appears deviated anteriorly, dislocated outside the septomarginal band, as to create infundibular stenosis and VSD (Fig. 11.15). Also the pulmonary valve may appear stenotic, and it is frequently bicuspid. The right-to-left shunt through the VSD, with blood flow partially forwarded from the right ventricle to the aorta, accounts for dextroposition of the aorta, its overriding across the ventricular septum and its biventricular origin, as well as for the systemic right ventricle with right ventricular hypertrophy. The complex (tetralogy of Fallot) may present frequently with associated lesions: right aortic arch, AV septal defect and anomalous coronary arteries.

The Blalock-Thomas-Taussig procedure, initially the only surgical treatment available for tetralogy of Fallot, was palliative but not curative. Total repair of

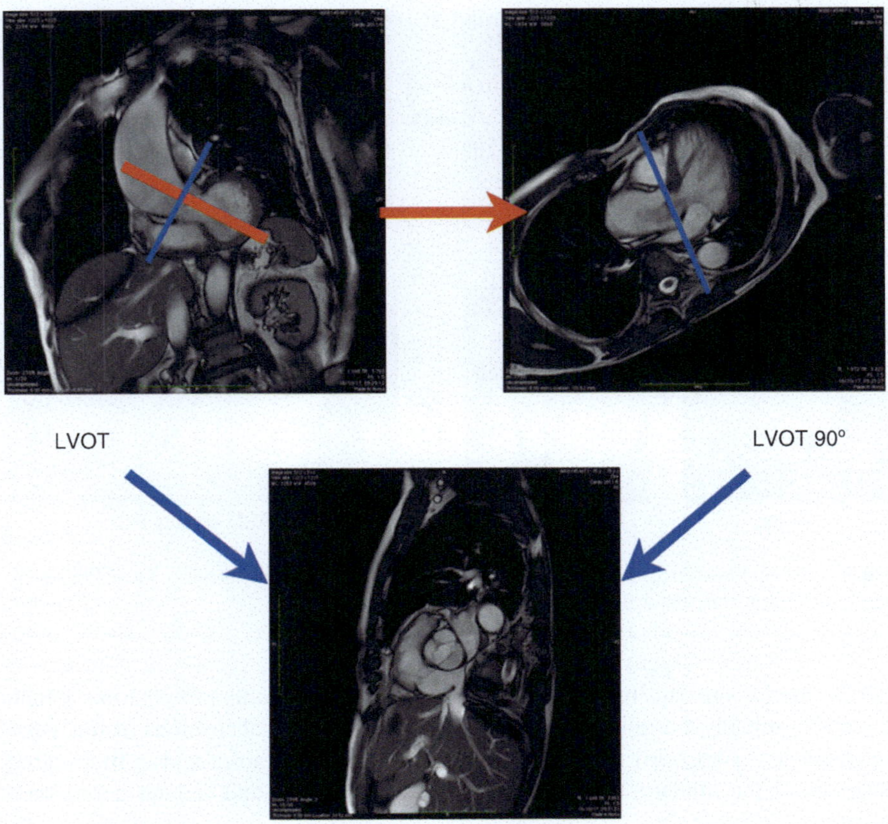

Fig. 11.13 Illustrative case of bicuspid aortic valve assessed by CMR

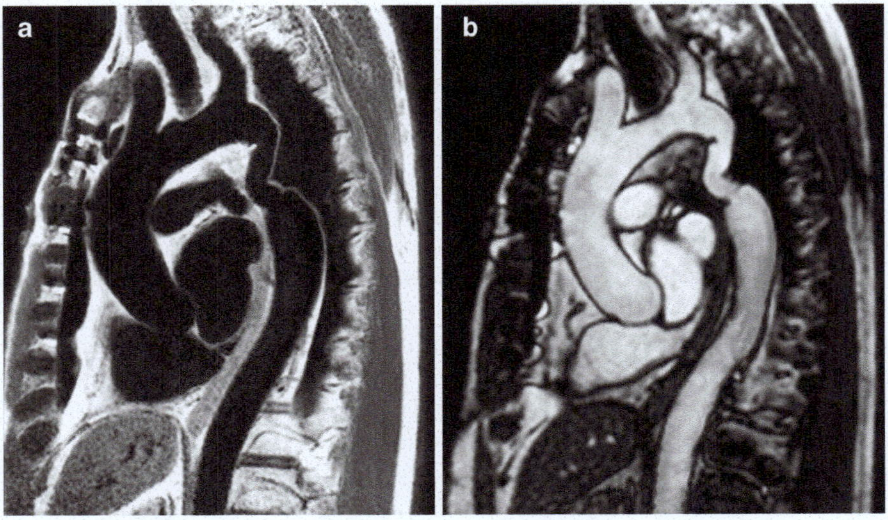

Fig. 11.14 Coarctation of the aorta: panel **a** shows a T1-weighted image for the morphological study, while panel **b** is a cine SSFP

Fig. 11.15 Tetralogy of Fallot

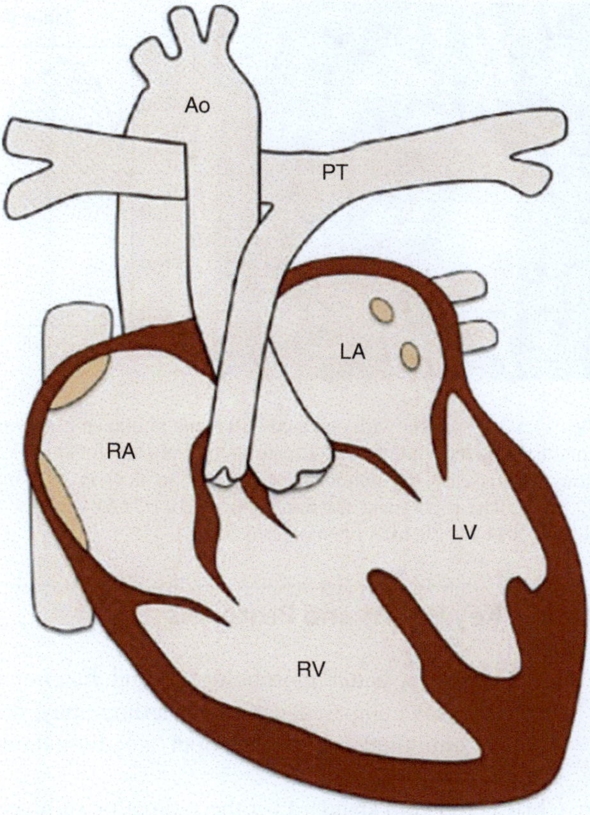

tetralogy of Fallot initially carried a high mortality risk, but this risk has gone down steadily over the years. Surgery is now often carried out in infants 1 year of age or younger with less than 5% perioperative mortality. The open-heart surgery is designed to relieve the right ventricular outflow tract stenosis by careful resection of the muscle to relieve RVOT obstruction and to repair VSD with a patch. Ninety percent of people with total repair as babies develop a progressively leaky pulmonary valve later in life. It is recommended that they follow up at a specialized adult congenital heart disease centre. CMR is very important to assess RV volumes and function as well as the degree of pulmonary regurgitation (a case example is reported in Fig. 11.16). A significant pulmonary regurgitation has a regurgitant fraction (RF) >35%. Pulmonary surgery is indicated before RV deterioration develops with a moderate to severe pulmonary regurgitation (RF > 25%) and RV telediastolic volume >150 mL/m^2. A reduced possibility of RV recovery can be predicted with RV telediastolic volume >160–170 mL/m^2 and RV telesystolic volume >82–85 mL/m^2 [10].

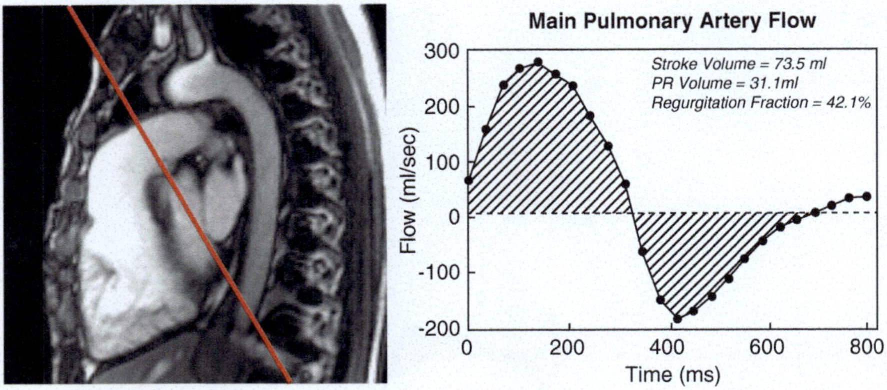

Fig. 11.16 A patient with operated Fallot and pulmonary regurgitation assessed by CMR. Phase contrast sequences allow to estimate the pulmonary forward flow and backward or regurgitant flow. In this case the pulmonary regurgitation flow is 31.1 mL, while RV stroke volume is 73.5 mL. The regurgitant fraction (RF) is (31.1/73.5) × 100 = 42% (from J Cardiovasc Magn Reson. 2011 Jan 20;13:9, open access)

11.4 Key Points and Protocols

- CMR allows a better morphological and functional evaluation of congenital heart diseases compared with echocardiography, due to the capability of performing unlimited sections without any limitation as for echocardiographic windows.
- CMR is the gold standard for the estimation of biventricular volumes and functions and especially for the study of right chambers.
- Specific CMR sequences for the study of congenital heart diseases include cine SSFP, phase contrast sequences for the study of flows and shunts and assessment of the ratio Qp/Qs.
- More common CHD in adults are atrial septal defects, bicuspid aortic valves, operated aortic coarctation, tetralogy of Fallot and corrected transposition of great arteries.
- CMR allows to evaluate the possible complications of surgical interventions for CHD and allows a careful follow-up of these patients.

References

1. Wood JC. Anatomical assessment of congenital heart disease. J Cardiovasc Magn Reson. 2006;8(4):595–606.
2. Fratz S, Hess J, Schuhbaeck A, Buchner C, Hendrich E, Martinoff S, Stern H. Routine clinical cardiovascular magnetic resonance in paediatric and adult congenital heart disease: patients, protocols, questions asked and contributions made. J Cardiovasc Magn Reson. 2008;10:46.

3. Ntsinjana HN, Hughes ML, Taylor AM. The role of cardiovascular magnetic resonance in pediatric congenital heart disease. J Cardiovasc Magn Reson. 2011;13:51.
4. Fratz S, Chung T, Greil GF, Samyn MM, Taylor AM, Valsangiacomo Buechel ER, Yoo SJ, Powell AJ. Guidelines and protocols for cardiovascular magnetic resonance in children and adults with congenital heart disease: SCMR expert consensus group on congenital heart disease. J Cardiovasc Magn Reson. 2013;15:51.
5. Kramer CM, Barkhausen J, Flamm SD, Kim RJ, Nagel E, Society for Cardiovascular Magnetic Resonance Board of Trustees Task Force on Standardized Protocols. Standardized cardiovascular magnetic resonance (CMR) protocols 2013 update. J Cardiovasc Magn Reson. 2013;15:91.
6. Schrot J, Pietila T, Sahu A. State of the art: 3D printing for creating compliant patient-specific congenital heart defect models. J Cardiovasc Magn Reson. 2014;16(Suppl 1):W19.
7. Dyverfeldt P, Bissell M, Barker AJ, Bolger AF, Carlhäll CJ, Ebbers T, Francios CJ, Frydrychowicz A, Geiger J, Giese D, Hope MD, Kilner PJ, Kozerke S, Myerson S, Neubauer S, Wieben O, Markl M. 4D flow cardiovascular magnetic resonance consensus statement. J Cardiovasc Magn Reson. 2015;17:72.
8. Thiene G, Frescura C. Anatomical and pathophysiological classification of congenital heart disease. Cardiovasc Pathol. 2010;19(5):259–74.
9. Herzog B, Kidambi A, Ballard G. Congenital Heart Disease Pocket Guide. Disponibile gratuitamente online all'indirizzo. https://www.escardio.org/Sub-specialty-communities/European-Association-of-Cardiovascular-Imaging-(EACVI)/Research-and-Publications/CMR-Pocket-Guides.
10. Geva T. Repaired tetralogy of Fallot: the roles of cardiovascular magnetic resonance in evaluating pathophysiology and for pulmonary valve replacement decision support. J Cardiovasc Magn Reson. 2011;13:9.

Aortic and Vascular Diseases

12

Contents

12.1 Introduction

CMR allows optimal visualization of the aorta and its pathological processes without the use of ionizing radiation and also without contrast agents if a MR angiography is not required [1–3]. Nevertheless it is not suitable for unstable patients and in emergency/urgency settings, such as for the study of aortic dissection.

In physiological conditions, the aortic root does not exceed 40 mm in men (Fig. 12.1) and progressively reduces its diameter distally (the superior limit of normality for the aortic root is 40 mm in men and 34 mm in women). Aging is responsible of a progressive increase in the dimensions of the aorta either in men (0.9 mm for each decade) or women (0.7 mm/10 years). Ideally, aortic diameter measures should be evaluated in short axis and telediastole (Fig. 12.2). There is no general agreement on the issue of inclusion or not of the aortic wall (especially for abdominal aortic aneurysms, the aortic walls are included in the measure of the size).

Other imaging techniques for the evaluation of the aorta include transthoracic echocardiography (allows especially the evaluation of the aortic valve, aortic root and proximal ascending aorta), transesophageal echocardiography (for the evaluation of ascending and descending aorta and acute aortic diseases), abdominal echography (for the evaluation of abdominal aneurysms) and CT (allows complete assessment of the aorta with also its calcification but requires the use of ionizing radiations).

M. Imazio et al., *Learning Cardiac Magnetic Resonance*,
https://doi.org/10.1007/978-3-030-11608-8_12

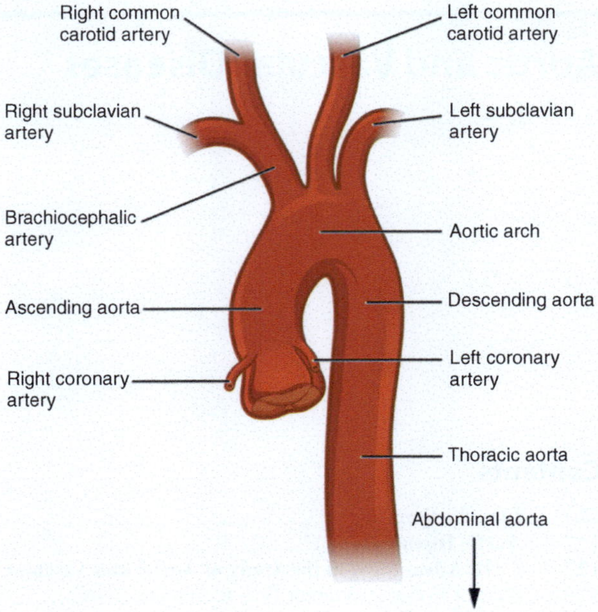

Fig. 12.1 Terminology of different sections of the aorta. From Wikimedia Commons

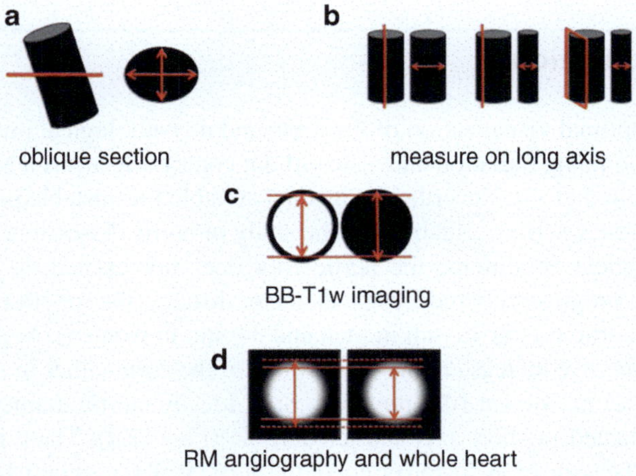

Fig. 12.2 Issues in aortic diameter measurements: possibility to overestimate the diameter (if measures are not taken perpendicularly to the flow direction due to an oblique section of the vessel; see panel **a**) or underestimate the diameter (measures on long axis of the diameter instead of short axis of the vessel; see panel **b**). In black-blood T1w imaging, measures may overestimate the diameter if the vessel wall is included (Panel **c**). In angiographic sequences, measure errors may also occur due to low spatial resolution, movement artefacts and lack of cardiac synchronization (Panel **d**). In 3D whole heart cardiosynchronization is present, but motion artefacts and low resolution may affect the measure.

12.2 Aortic Diseases

CMR is indicated for stable patients (Table 12.1); on this basis potentially unstable patients with a suspected or known acute aortic disease are evaluated by echocardiography and CT. In aortic dissection, patients are rarely evaluated by CMR for this reason (Fig. 12.3 and Table 12.2).

Cardiac RM allows an optimal visualization and measurement of aortic aneurysms at different levels also without contrast agent use. In the setting of suspected aortic bicuspid valve, CMR or CT may allow good morphological study of the valve and aortic size (especially useful to assess if the diameter is >50 mm or annual increase in size <3 mm) when echocardiography is not diagnostic (see also Table 12.3).

Table 12.1 Diagnostic value of different imaging techniques in the study of acute aortic syndromes

Lesion	TTE	TEE	TAC	RM
Ascending aorta dissection	++	+++	+++	+++
Aortic arch dissection	+	+	+++	+++
Evaluation of diameters	+	+++	+++	+++
Evaluation of mural thrombi	++	+++	+++	+++
Evaluation of intramural hematoma	+	+++	+++	+++
Evaluation of penetrating ulcer	+	+++	++	+++
Evaluation of involvement of collaterals	+	+	+++	+++

TTE transthoracic echocardiography, *TEE* transesophageal echocardiography

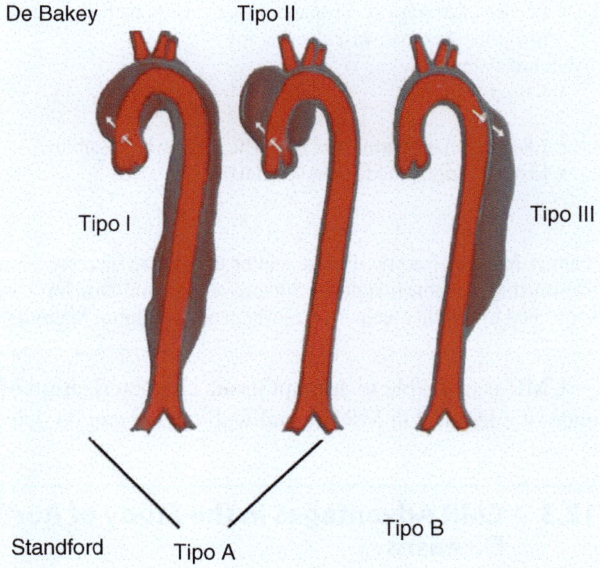

Fig. 12.3 Aortic dissection classification. From Wikimedia Commons

Table 12.2 Current indications to CMR in the evaluation of aortic disease

Recommendation	Class	LOE
Suspicion of an acute aortic syndrome in a stable patient	I	C
Repeated assessment of a patient with aortic dissection type B	I	C
Evaluation of the aortic root in bicuspid aortic valve by CT/CMR if echocardiography is not feasible/diagnostic	I	C
Evaluation of the aortic root in bicuspid aortic valve by CT/CMR to confirm aortic dilatation >50 mm or >3 mm/year.	I	C
Confirmation of chronic aortic disease by CT or CMR	I	C
Follow-up of young patients treated by endovascular interventions to avoid excessive exposure to ionizing radiation.	IIa	C

LOE level of evidence

Table 12.3 Cut-off values for the indication to intervention in aortic aneurysms according to 2014 ESC guidelines

Type and localization of the aneurysm	Diameter
Ascending aorta	
• Aortic root aneurysm in Marfan syndrome	≥50 mm (IC)
• Aortic root aneurysm in Marfan syndrome and risk factors[a]	≥45 mm (IIaC)
• Aortic root aneurysm and risk factors[a]	≥50 mm (IIaC)
• Aortic root aneurysm without elastopathy	≥55 mm (IIaC)
Aortic arch	
• Isolated aneurysm of the aortic arch	≥55 mm (IIaC)
Descending aorta	
• Endovascular treatment should be considered, rather than surgery, when anatomy is suitable	(IIaC)
• Endovascular treatment if diameter	≥55 mm (IIaC)
• If endovascular treatment if not possible, surgery should be indicated if diameter	≥60 mm (IIaC)
• In case of Marfan syndrome or other elastinopathies surgery is favourite over endovascular therapy	(IIaC)
Abdominal aorta	
• Surgery if	>55 mm or increasing >10 mm/year (IB)
• Endovascular treatment is favourite whenever possible	(IA o IC)
• Echocardiographic follow-up (IIaB)	30–39 mm (every 3 years) 40–44 mm (every 2 years) >44 mm (every year)

[a]Family history of aortic disease and/or aortic size increase >3 mm/year (on repeated measurements using the same imaging technique, at the same aorta level, with side-by-side comparison and confirmed by another technique), severe aortic or mitral regurgitation, or desire for pregnancy.

CMR is also able to attempt tissue characterization of the arterial wall (e.g. presence of edema). On MR arterial wall edema can be detected on STIR T2w images.

12.3 CMR Advantages in the Study of Aortic and Vascular Diseases

CMR is useful to assess the anatomy, morphology, size and tissue characterization of vessels (e.g. presence of edema in arteritis) without the use of ionizing radiations (Table 12.4). However, CMR requires a stable patient and cannot be performed in

Table 12.4 Comparison of different imaging techniques for the study of the aorta

Advantages/limitations	TTE	TEE	CT	MR	Angiography
Easy-to-use	+++	++	+++	++	+
Reliability	+	+++	+++	+++	++
Bedside/urgent use	++	++	–	–	++
Possibility of serial studies	++	+	++	++	–
Study of arterial walls	+	+++	+++	+++	–
Costs	+	+	++	+++	+++
Exposure to ionizing radiations	0	0	+++	0	+++
Risk of nephrotoxicity	0	0	+++	–	+++

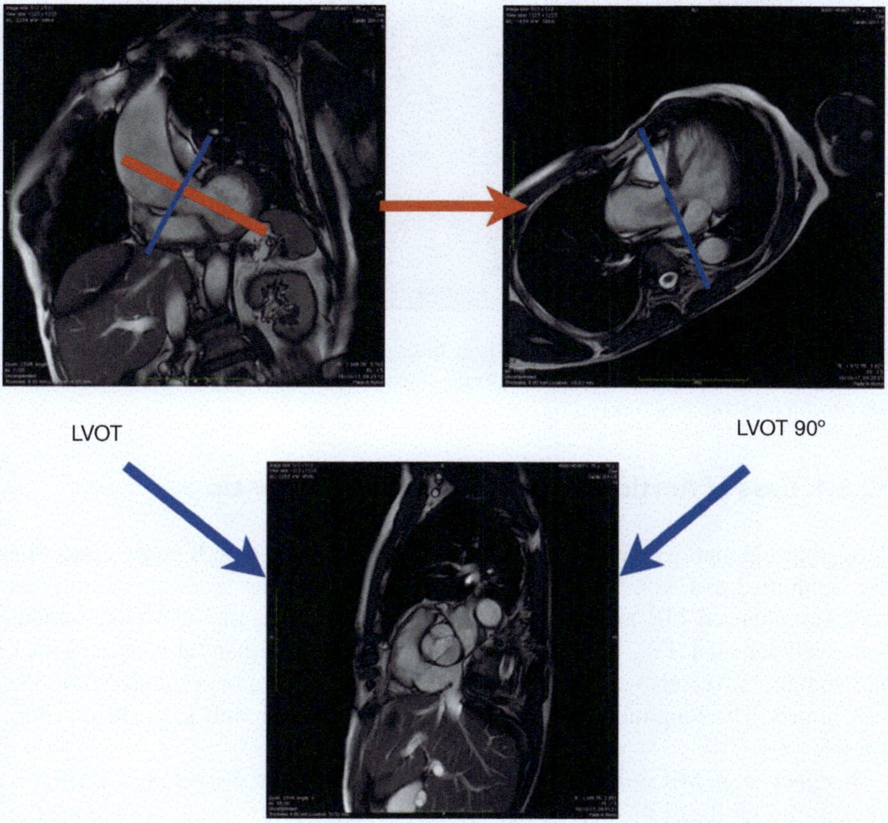

Fig. 12.4 Assessment of the aortic root and aortic valve morphology (case of bicuspid valve)

emergency/urgency. Moreover the exam is less available than other imaging techniques and more time-consuming. It is also possible to perform RM angiography by contrast injection and 3D reconstruction as in CT. Tissue characterization of the vessel wall is possible in arteritis by detection of aortic wall edema and LGE (when contrast agents are used). A specific limitation of CMR is the inability to study calcifications such as in CT. Aortic measures are performed in cine imaging as telediastolic diameters using short axis views that should be perpendicular to blood flow (for aortic root measures a short axis is taken from LVOT and VOT 90°; see Fig. 12.4).

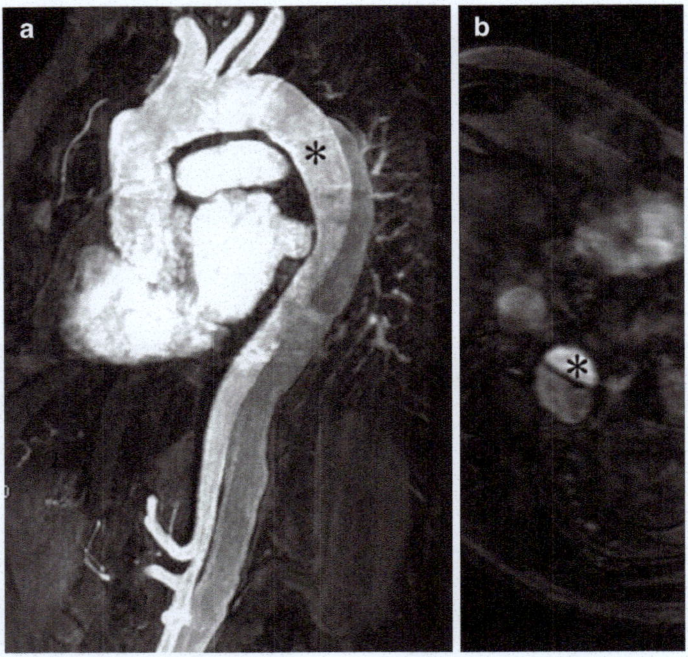

Fig. 12.5 CEMRA imaging of a case of type B aortic dissection. The true lumen is contrast enhanced (see white asterisk), and it is smaller than the false lumen (see panel **a** for long-axis view and panel **b** for short-axis view)

12.3.1 Case of Aortic Dissection Type B on Follow-Up

A 67-year-old man with arterial hypertension and a known type B aortic dissection was submitted to CMR as a follow-up control study of the aortic dissection. On contrast-enhanced MR angiography (CEMRA) sequences, true and false lumens were well depicted (Fig. 12.5). The true lumen was smaller than false, and the neck and abdominal vessels were not involved in the dissection and originated from the true lumen. The longitudinal extension of dissection was well seen till the iliac arteries.

In conclusion, MR images confirmed stable type B aortic dissection. CEMRA is most useful for the evaluation of the location, extent, diameters and involvement of branch vessels of the aorta.

12.4 Key Points and Protocols

- CMR allows the morphological study and assessment of size of each segment of the aorta (main advantages).
- T2-weighted imaging may allow to detect wall edema for the study of suspected arteritis (additional advantage).

- Main limitations of MR are the need for stable patients, inability to study calcifications, long processing times, more limited availability and higher costs than echocardiography and CT.
- A standard MR protocol for the evaluation of chronic aortic disease includes cine sequences, T1w imaging for morphological study, T2w imaging and LGE for assessment of wall inflammation. MR angiography and 3D reconstruction may be required for specific cases.

References

1. Erbel R, Aboyans V, Boileau C, Bossone E, Bartolomeo RD, Eggebrecht H, Evangelista A, Falk V, Frank H, Gaemperli O, Grabenwöger M, Haverich A, Iung B, Manolis AJ, Meijboom F, Nienaber CA, Roffi M, Rousseau H, Sechtem U, Sirnes PA, Allmen RS, Vrints CJ, ESC Committee for Practice Guidelines. 2014 ESC Guidelines on the diagnosis and treatment of aortic diseases: document covering acute and chronic aortic diseases of the thoracic and abdominal aorta of the adult. The Task Force for the Diagnosis and Treatment of Aortic Diseases of the European Society of Cardiology (ESC). Eur Heart J. 2014;35(41):2873–926.
2. Kramer CM, Barkhausen J, Flamm SD, Kim RJ, Nagel E, Society for Cardiovascular Magnetic Resonance Board of Trustees Task Force on Standardized Protocols. Standardized cardiovascular magnetic resonance (CMR) protocols 2013 update. J Cardiovasc Magn Reson. 2013;15:91.
3. Dyverfeldt P, Bissell M, Barker AJ, Bolger AF, Carlhäll CJ, Ebbers T, Francios CJ, Frydrychowicz A, Geiger J, Giese D, Hope MD, Kilner PJ, Kozerke S, Myerson S, Neubauer S, Wieben O, Markl M. 4D flow cardiovascular magnetic resonance consensus statement. J Cardiovasc Magn Reson. 2015;17:72. https://doi.org/10.1186/s12968-015-0174-5.

CMR and Devices

13

Contents

Pacemakers and implantable cardiac defibrillators, together usually considered as "cardiac implantable electronic devices" (CIEDs), have been traditionally considered contraindications for cardiac magnetic resonance (CMR) also in previous guidelines [1–3].

Nevertheless it is estimated that 50–75% of patients with CIEDs will develop an indication for CMR due to comorbidities during their lifetime after device implantation, and, in specific cases, CMR is essential for their appropriate management. On this basis, a review of the potential effects of the CMR on the implanted devices is necessary.

13.1 CMR Effects on Implanted Devices

The CMR system has three major components that may affect an implanted device: (1) the main static magnetic field, (2) gradient fields, and (3) radiofrequencies.

A summary of the main possible effects of each component on implanted devices is reported in Table 13.1.

All the three components have the potential to interact with the device altering its normal function; radiofrequencies have also the potentiality to induce case and especially leads heating since pacing leads may act as antennae concentrating electromagnetic energy at tips, which can lead to heating of the surrounding tissue and cause tissue damage with edema and/or fibrosis. This could be responsible for

M. Imazio et al., *Learning Cardiac Magnetic Resonance*,
https://doi.org/10.1007/978-3-030-11608-8_13

Table 13.1 Potential effects of CMT components on implanted devices

Potential effect	Main fields (static)	Gradient fields	Radiofrequency
Force and torque	X		
Vibration	X	X	
Device interaction[a]	X	X	X
Case heating		X	X
Lead heating			X
Myocardial stimulation		X	X

[a]Possible damage and interference with normal function

increased pacing thresholds, loss of capture and in more severe cases up to perforation. In animal models in pigs, the electrode tips had an increased temperature of up to 20 °C in the setting of a SAR approaching 3.8 W/kg that is higher than in routine CMR scan. Modern MR conditional pacing leads have altered diameter and materials so that it remains inert at the resonant frequency.

Since PMs and ICDs contain ferromagnetic material, they are subject to force and torque effects by the main magnetic field. Modern CIEDs, which have been manufactured after the year 2000, have reduced ferromagnetic content and appear safe in the CMR 1.5 T environment after 4 to 6 weeks from implantation [4–7]. According to European guidelines [7], a minimal 6 weeks time is required following implantation to allow sufficient anchorage of the device. Modern pacing leads are constructed with materials that are less magnetically susceptible and have a very little risk of movement or dislodgement if connected to the generator case.

The greatest risk is especially for devices manufactured before the year 2000 (so-called "legacy devices"), while hardware and software changes have reduced the risk for the newer devices although a specific distinction should be made for MR conditional devices versus non-MR conditional devices (see later in the chapter).

Potential causes of malfunction in older devices included: (1) *reed switches activation* in the magnetic field, (2) *electrical reset*, (3) *inappropriate pacing and inhibition of therapies by radiofrequencies*, and (4) *ICD battery depletion and damage*.

Reed switches are electrical switches operated by an applied magnetic field that were generally incorporated to allow device interrogation. The magnet application allowed the *reed switch activation* inhibiting demand functions and usually setting the device to an asynchronous mode. Thus variable reed switch responses have been demonstrated with a device in a MR scan inducing asynchronous pacing (risk of R on T phenomenon and induction of arrhythmias) and transient or continuous loss of pacing (risk of asystole in pacemaker-dependent patients). In ICDs the activation of the reed switch is commonly responsible for the deactivation of therapies. In MR-conditional devices, reed switches have been replaced by a solid state or hall sensor.

Electrical reset or *power on reset* is an emergency/backup mode that allows a PM to revert to a VVI pacing mode at a lower rate limit with all advanced functions turned off at the end of the battery life. For ICDs it is a safety mechanism that prevents inappropriate shocks from a damaged device (it is essentially a VVI backup mode with no therapies). ICD cannot be reprogrammed and the device should be replaced. In PM-dependent patients without an underlying ventricular rhythm, the conversion of an asynchronous pacing to VVI mode with radiofrequency pulses wrongly interpreted by intrinsic electrical activity by the PM has been advocated as a cause of severe incidents with deaths in older case reports.

Radiofrequency pulses may be responsible for *inappropriate pacing and inhibition of therapies* (e.g. asynchronous pacing, programming changes and battery depletion can also be wrongly interpreted by spontaneous electrical activity by PMs).

ICDs cannot charge the capacitor in a MR environment, and multiple attempts to charge the capacitor may lead to *ICD battery depletion and damage*.

Although older reports of isolated incidents in patients with non-MR conditional devices including asystole, ventricular fibrillation and death, more recent reports after 2010 have shown no casualties and limited effects.

In addition to safety issues, PMs and ICDs are responsible for significant distortion of the magnetic field homogeneity and thus artefacts that may affect the image quality (see later in the chapter).

In a recent review on >1400 CMR exams in patients with pacemakers from 15 studies, no deaths were reported [8]. In another study (prospective and non-randomized) involving 438 patients with devices (54% with pacemakers and 46% with defibrillators) who underwent 555 MRI studies (40% brain, 22% spine, 16% heart, 13% abdominal and 9% extremities), limited effects were noted. In three patients (0.7%), the device reverted to a transient backup programming mode without long-term effects. In addition, minor changes in atrial and ventricular lead impedance were seen, but no significant changes in pacing capture thresholds were noted. Pacing mode was changed to asynchronous for pacemaker-dependent patients and to demand for others. Tachyarrhythmia functions were disabled. Blood pressure, electrocardiography, oximetry and symptoms were monitored by a nurse with experience in cardiac life support and device programming who had immediate backup from an electrophysiologist [9]. In the MagnaSafe Registry, a multicenter, prospective cohort study of up to 1500 MRI examinations in patients with non-MR conditional pacemakers or implantable cardioverter-defibrillators implanted after 2001 who undergo clinically indicated nonthoracic MRI following a specific protocol to ensure that preventable potential adverse events are mitigated, no severe adverse events occurred as well as device or lead failure [10, 11]. Patients underwent clinically indicated nonthoracic MRI at 1.5 tesla, were appropriately screened and had the device reprogrammed in accordance with the prespecified protocol. If the patient was asymptomatic and had an intrinsic heart rate of at least 40 beats per minute, the device was programmed to a no-pacing mode (ODO or OVO). Symptomatic patients or those with an intrinsic heart rate of less than 40 beats per minute were determined to be pacing-dependent, and the device was reprogrammed to an asynchronous pacing mode (DOO or VOO). For non-pacing-dependent patients with an ICD, all bradycardia and tachycardia therapies were inactivated before the MRI. Pacing-dependent patients with an ICD were excluded, because not all ICD models allowed for independent inactivation of tachycardia and bradycardia therapies. After the MRI, baseline settings were restored, full device interrogation was repeated and, if necessary, the device was reprogrammed to maintain adequate pacing and sensing.

On this basis, CMR scanning in patients with non-MR conditional devices should be carefully evaluated and requires adequate monitoring with pre- and post-examination check and reprogramming of the devices.

13.2 Image Quality in Patients with Implanted Devices

PMs and ICDs are responsible of possible significant distortions of the magnetic field due to their ferromagnetic content [12]. The ferromagnetic content of the devices creates magnetic field inhomogeneities that alter MR signal and produces artefacts (*metal susceptibility artefacts*).

These metal susceptibility artefacts may appear as bright or dark bands due to either misregistration or signal loss (Fig. 13.1). Artefact size depends on the volume and ferromagnetic properties of the device but also the direction and strength of the magnetic field gradient as well as the type of MR sequence. MR sequences with the greatest sensitivity to magnetic field inhomogeneities include the balanced steady-state free precession (bSSFP) sequences and inversion recovery sequences and those with fast K-space acquisition (e.g. EPI and spiral mode). Gradient-echo

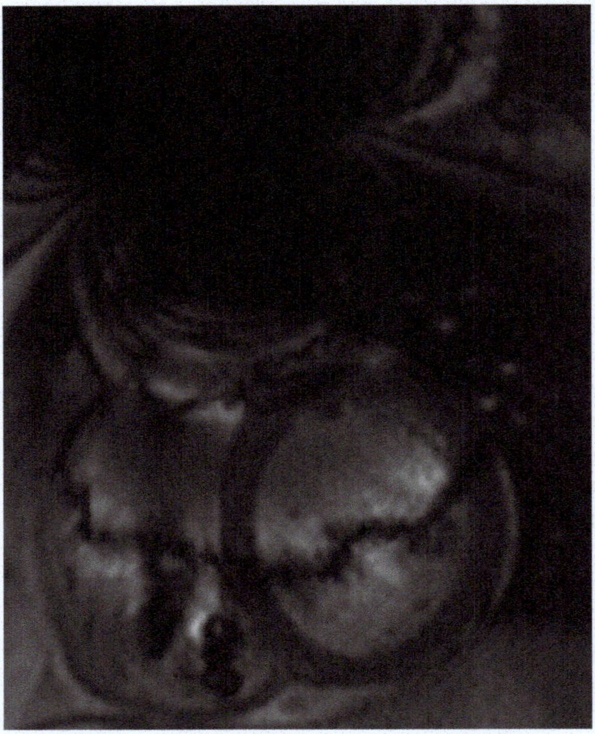

Fig. 13.1 A metal susceptibility artefact in a patient with an implanted device. Artefacts appear as bright or dark bands due to either misregistration or signal loss

sequences are affected by a degree that is largely dependent on TE setting: a short TE allows less time for dephasing and limits signal loss. Spin-echo sequences are less prone to these artefacts.

The utility of CMR in patients with left-sided ICD/BiV-ICD systems may be limited because of larger PM/ICD artefacts than in patients with PM or right-sided ICD/BiV-ICD systems.

13.3 MR Conditional and Non-MR Conditional Devices

MR conditional devices are implanted devices that are safe under specific conditions that are declared by the manufacturer. All the components of the device (generator and leads) should be MR conditional to allow safe MR under specific conditions (follow the manufacturer instructions). Usually the static field strength limit is 1.5 T, SAR limit is 2 W/Kg and slew rate is <200 T/m/s.

Industries have made significant changes in both hardware and software of devices to allow reduced interferences of the device with the MR environment (Table 13.2).

In any case a device interrogation is mandatory before and after the MR scan. Before the examination, "MR safe" mode is activated (usually asynchronous pacing is programmed without sensing to reduce the risk of electromagnetic interferences), and advanced functions are switched off. Some MR conditional devices have increased pacing stimulus to minimize the risk of loss of capture.

Non-MR conditional devices are implantable devices that have not been tested to be safe under prespecified conditions. Scanning patients with these devices is off-label and although not absolutely contraindicated should be performed only if there are compelling indications for MR and no other diagnostic alternatives under well-monitored conditions and with a pre- and post-examination check and reprogramming of the device.

The US guidelines for safe MR scanning strongly discourage MR in patients that are PM-dependent or have ICDs and discourage MR of non-MR conditional PM in patients that are no PM dependent, except in case of urgent need [1].

The justification for such restrictions is related to the unpredictability of electromagnetical interferences with the devices and the need for a special care in screening, monitoring and post-examination check and reprogramming of devices to minimize the risks for patients. According to the American College of Radiology,

Table 13.2 Hardware and software changes in MR conditional implantable devices

Hardware	
Generator	Reduction of ferromagnetic material Replacement of reed switch with solid state technology (e.g. Hall sensor) Bandstop filter at 64 MHz for case to shield the generator
Leads	Changes in the design to alter the resonant frequency of the lead Bandstop filter at 64 MHz at lead tip in some leads
Software	Dedicated MRI pacing mode for the duration of the scan

the following clinical indications have the highest rating for MRI (8 or 9): chronic neck pain (normal radiograms with neurological signs and symptoms), low back pain in patients older than 70 years, soft tissue masses, stroke symptoms and possible or probable Alzheimer's disease.

13.4 European Guidelines on MRI in Patients with Implanted Devices

European guidelines on magnetic resonance imaging (MRI) in patients with implanted cardiac devices were issued in 2013 [7]. European guidelines recognize that potential adverse effects of MRI on implanted devices include radiofrequency-induced heating of lead tips, pacing inhibition/dysfunction, asynchronous pacing with the possible induction of arrhythmias, transient reed switch activation, change of programmation and capture threshold. The closer the scanning area is to the device, the higher is the risk for the patient. Initial experience on 0.5 T and subsequent 1.5 T MR scan suggest that MRI can be safely performed if specific precautions are adopted. Nevertheless ICDs and the majority of PMs (all non-MR conditional devices) are considered contraindications to MRI by the Food and Drug Administration (FDA). The European Society of Cardiology (ESC) guidelines recommend careful screening of implanted devices with pre-scan programming, monitoring during scan and post-scan reprogramming. For conventional PM/ICD (non-MR conditional), a MRI scan at 1.5 T can be performed with a low risk of complication if the management algorithm reported in Fig. 13.2 is followed

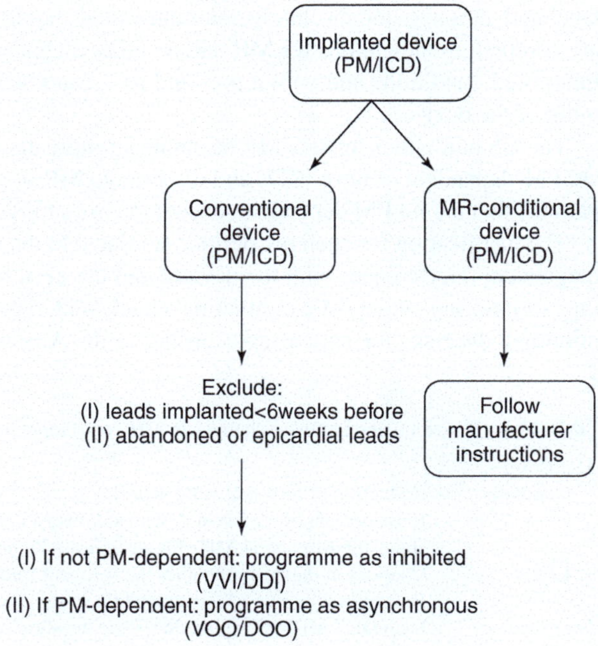

Fig. 13.2 Management flow chart for patients with implanted devices (PM/ICD) undergoing MRI for compelling indications according to ESC guidelines. See text for additional explanations

(recommendation Class IIb, LOE B). In such patients the presence of leads implanted <6 weeks before the possible MRI and abandoned or epicardial leads should be excluded (increased risk of RF-induced heating of leads). Then if the patient is non-PM dependent, the device should be programmed as VVI/DDI (inhibited). If the patient is PM dependent, the device should be programmed as VOO/DOO (asynchronous). Other pacing functions and monitoring as well as ATP/shock therapies (ICD) should be deactivated. During MRI a close ECG and symptom monitoring is warranted. After the MRI scan, the device should be rechecked and reprogrammed.

For MR conditional devices, MRI at 1.5 T can be performed safely following the manufacturer instructions (recommendation Class IIa, LOE B).

References

1. Levine GN, Gomes AS, Arai AE, Bluemke DA, Flamm SD, Kanal E, Manning WJ, Martin ET, Smith JM, Wilke N, Shellock FS, American Heart Association Committee on Diagnostic and Interventional Cardiac Catheterization; American Heart Association Council on Clinical Cardiology; American Heart Association Council on Cardiovascular Radiology and Intervention. Safety of magnetic resonance imaging in patients with cardiovascular devices: an American Heart Association scientific statement from the Committee on Diagnostic and Interventional Cardiac Catheterization, Council on Clinical Cardiology, and the Council. Circulation. 2007;116(24):2878–91.
2. Jung W, Jäckle S, Zvereva V. MRI and implantable cardiac electronic devices. Curr Opin Cardiol. 2015;30(1):65–73.
3. Yee R, Verma A, Beardsall M, Fraser J, Philippon F, Exner DV. Canadian Cardiovascular Society/Canadian Heart Rhythm Society joint position statement on the use of remote monitoring for cardiovascular implantable electronic device follow-up. Can J Cardiol. 2013;29(6):644–51.
4. Lowe MD, Plummer CJ, Manisty CH, Linker NJ, British Heart Rhythm Society. Safe use of MRI in people with cardiac implantable electronic devices. Heart. 2015;101(24):1950–3.
5. Nordbeck P, Ertl G, Ritter O. Magnetic resonance imaging safety in pacemaker and implantable cardioverter defibrillator patients: how far have we come? Eur Heart J. 2015;36(24):1505–11.
6. Miller JD, Nazarian S, Halperin HR. Implantable electronic cardiac devices and compatibility with magnetic resonance imaging. J Am Coll Cardiol. 2016;68(14):1590–8.
7. Brignole M, Auricchio A, Baron-Esquivias G, Bordachar P, Boriani G, Breithardt OA, Cleland J, Deharo JC, Delgado V, Elliott PM, Gorenek B, Israel CW, Leclercq C, Linde C, Mont L, Padeletti L, Sutton R, Vardas PE, ESC Committee for Practice Guidelines (CPG), Zamorano JL, Achenbach S, Baumgartner H, Bax JJ, Bueno H, Dean V, Deaton C, Erol C, Fagard R, Ferrari R, Hasdai D, Hoes AW, Kirchhof P, Knuuti J, Kolh P, Lancellotti P, Linhart A, Nihoyannopoulos P, Piepoli MF, Ponikowski P, Sirnes PA, Tamargo JL, Tendera M, Torbicki A, Wijns W, Windecker S, Document Reviewers, Kirchhof P, Blomstrom-Lundqvist C, Badano LP, Aliyev F, Bänsch D, Baumgartner H, Bsata W, Buser P, Charron P, Daubert JC, Dobreanu D, Faerestrand S, Hasdai D, Hoes AW, Le Heuzey JY, Mavrakis H, McDonagh T, Merino JL, Nawar MM, Nielsen JC, Pieske B, Poposka L, Ruschitzka F, Tendera M, Van Gelder IC, Wilson CM. 2013 ESC Guidelines on cardiac pacing and cardiac resynchronization therapy: the Task Force on cardiac pacing and resynchronization therapy of the European Society of Cardiology (ESC). Developed in collaboration with the European Heart Rhythm Association (EHRA). Eur Heart J. 2013;34(29):2281–329.
8. Zikria JF, Machnicki S, Rhim E, Bhatti T, Graham RE. MRI of patients with cardiac pacemakers: a review of the medical literature. AJR Am J Roentgenol. 2011;196(2):390–401.

9. Nazarian S, Hansford R, Roguin A, Goldsher D, Zviman MM, Lardo AC, Caffo BS, Frick KD, Kraut MA, Kamel IR, Calkins H, Berger RD, Bluemke DA, Halperin HR. A prospective evaluation of a protocol for magnetic resonance imaging of patients with implanted cardiac devices. Ann Intern Med. 2011;155(7):415–24.
10. Russo RJ. Determining the risks of clinically indicated nonthoracic magnetic resonance imaging at 1.5 T for patients with pacemakers and implantable cardioverter-defibrillators: rationale and design of the MagnaSafe Registry. Am Heart J. 2013;165(3):266–72.
11. Russo RJ, Costa HS, Silva PD, Anderson JL, Arshad A, Biederman RW, Boyle NG, Frabizzio JV, Birgersdotter-Green U, Higgins SL, Lampert R, Machado CE, Martin ET, Rivard AL, Rubenstein JC, Schaerf RH, Schwartz JD, Shah DJ, Tomassoni GF, Tominaga GT, Tonkin AE, Uretsky S, Wolff SD. Assessing the risks associated with MRI in patients with a pacemaker or defibrillator. N Engl J Med. 2017;376(8):755–64.
12. Sasaki T, Hansford R, Zviman MM, Kolandaivelu A, Bluemke DA, Berger RD, Calkins H, Halperin HR, Nazarian S. Quantitative assessment of artifacts on cardiac magnetic resonance imaging of patients with pacemakers and implantable cardioverter-defibrillators. Circ Cardiovasc Imaging. 2011;4(6):662–70.

Common Artefacts

14

Contents

14.1 Overview

An artefact is a finding on MR images that is not real, but it is produced incidentally by the use of specific techniques and sequences [1]. CMR is prone to artefacts since it is depicting a moving organ because of cardiac contractions, breathing and blood flows but also because of different tissue characteristics (fat, muscle, blood) and possible presence of devices [1, 2].

An artefact may affect the quality of the images and reduce diagnostic capabilities. Knowledge of artefacts that are generated during the acquisition process is important to make corrections and reduce the negative impact of artefacts on the quality of the CMR exam [3, 4]. This appendix will provide a brief overview of artefacts in CMR imaging. The main artefacts that can be encountered in CMR include:

1. Movement artefacts (breathing, cardiac, flow-related)
2. Truncation artefacts (Gibbs ringing)

M. Imazio et al., *Learning Cardiac Magnetic Resonance*,
https://doi.org/10.1007/978-3-030-11608-8_14

3. Aliasing artefacts
4. Chemical-shift artefacts
5. Magnetic field inhomogeneity artefacts

14.2 Movement Artefacts

14.2.1 Ghosting (Breathing Motion Artefacts)

Breathing motion artefacts are usually caused by the inability of patients to keep breath-holding. Such artefacts are classically represented by doubling of imaging contours with evident movement of the thorax (Fig. 14.1).

Possible solutions are keeping end-inspiration breath-holding instead of expiratory breath-holding, the use of single-shot imaging, low-resolution imaging to reduce acquisition times and thus breath-holding. Additional options include the use of sequences with the use of navigators to follow diaphragm movements (to guide the acquisition of images in a specific phase but prolonging the overall time of image acquisition) or the use of real-time imaging with free breathing.

14.2.2 Cardiac Motion Artefacts

Cardiac synchronization by ECG monitoring allows to acquire images during a specific phase of cardiac cycle when the heart is relatively still (mesodiastole). However, such synchronization can be lost or difficult in case of arrhythmias or bad-quality ECG signal producing cardiac motion artefacts that appear as faded borders (Fig. 14.2).

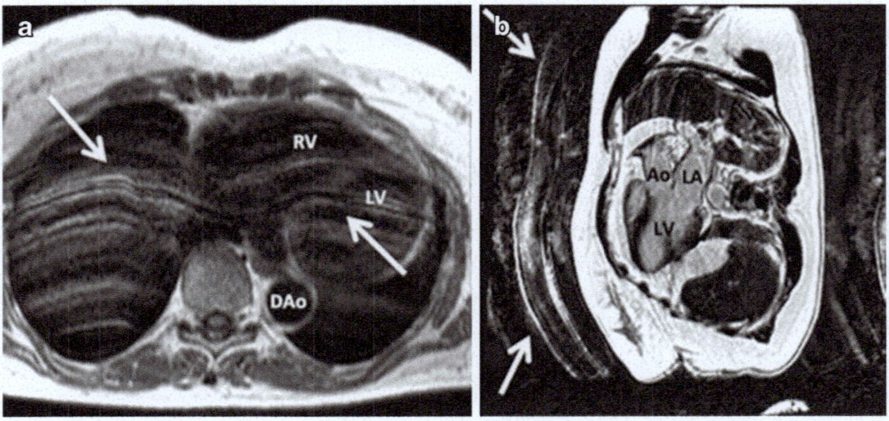

Fig. 14.1 Breathing motion artefacts (ghosting; see white lines). From Ferreira et al. Journal of Cardiovascular Magnetic Resonance 2013, 15:41. Open access

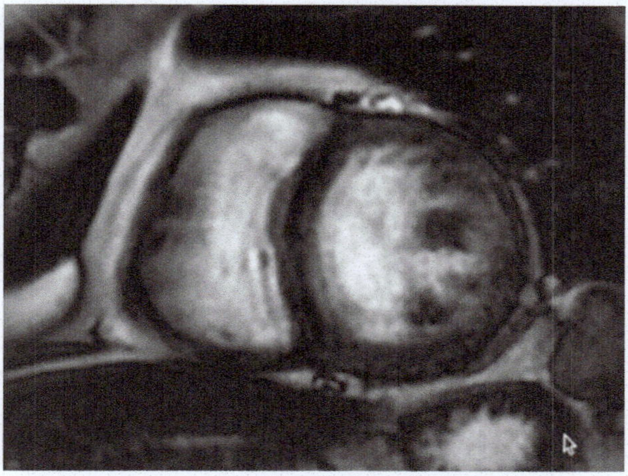

Fig. 14.2 Cardiac artefacts with fading cardiac borders due to impaired cardiosynchronization by frequent premature ventricular beats. Short-axis image of ventricles

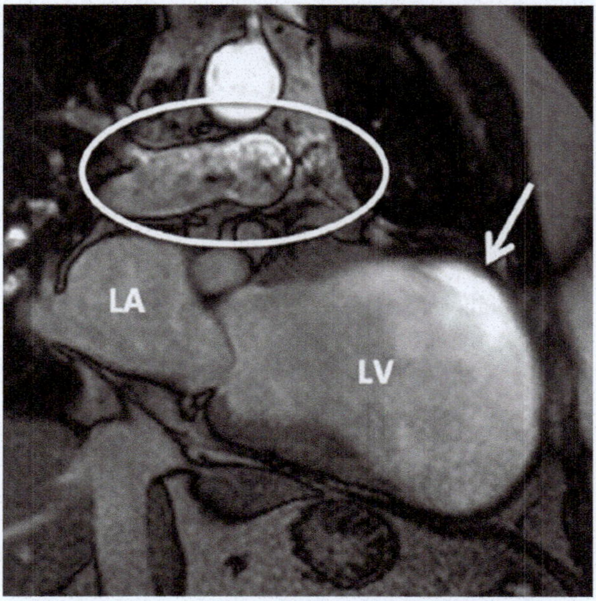

Fig. 14.3 Flow motion artefact in pulmonary artery trunk with accelerated flow. From Ferreira et al. Journal of Cardiovascular Magnetic Resonance 2013, 15:41. Open access

This artefact can be attenuated by the use of the function "arrhythmia rejection" that allows to exclude images acquired during irregular RR times or alternatively by real-time acquisition at the expenses of a lower spatial resolution.

14.2.3 Flow Artefacts

In case of high velocity flows of blood, the homogeneity of magnetization can be impaired in SSFP cine imaging. This artefact is typically seen in outflow tracts of ventricles or great arteries (Fig. 14.3).

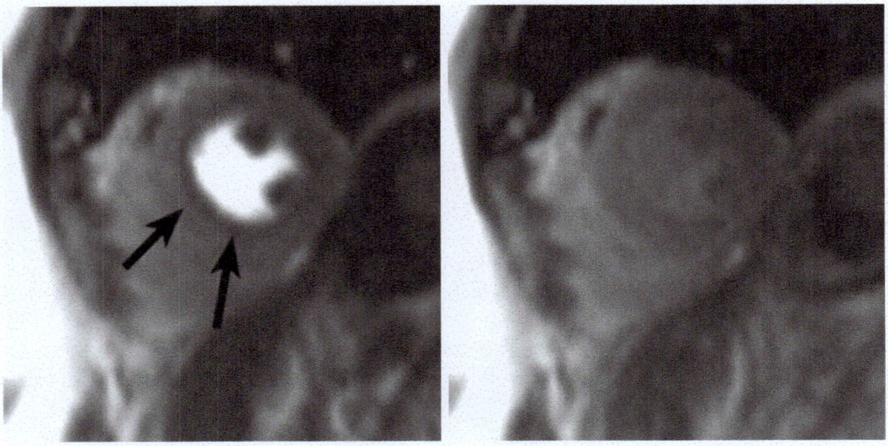

Fig. 14.4 Dark rim artefact in perfusion study (panels **d** and **e**) and cine imaging (panel **f**). From Ferreira et al. Journal of Cardiovascular Magnetic Resonance 2013, 15:41

14.3 Truncation Artefacts (Gibbs Ringing)

Truncation artefacts (also named Gibbs ringing) are produced whenever there is a border or interface between tissues with different signal intensity (for CMR typically blood/wall interface). It is caused by a specific limitation of Fourier transform to elaborate sudden changes of signal frequencies. In CMR, Gibbs ringing is often seen in perfusion studies at the endocardial border and may mimic a subendocardial perfusion defect (Fig. 14.4). This artefact is also known as "dark rim artefact". Dark rim artefact can be distinguished from a real perfusion defect by different features: the artefact defect appears before the arrival of contrast media in the LV cavity, and it lasts few heartbeats and has a limited extension. It can be reduced by increasing spatial resolution at the expenses of a longer acquisition time.

14.4 Aliasing Artefacts

It is a rather common artefact in CMR. This artefact occurs whenever the size of the object being imaged exceeds the field of view (FOV) in the phase-encode direction, the outside regions are wrapped into the opposite edge of the FOV (Fig. 14.5). Possible solutions are to increase the FOV and the use of saturation bands to suppress signals outside the FOV.

In phase contrast imaging, aliasing can occur when preselected maximal velocity (VENC) is lower than the real flow velocity (Fig. 14.6). Eco-Doppler data from echocardiography should be used as a guide to select the appropriate maximal velocity to be selected.

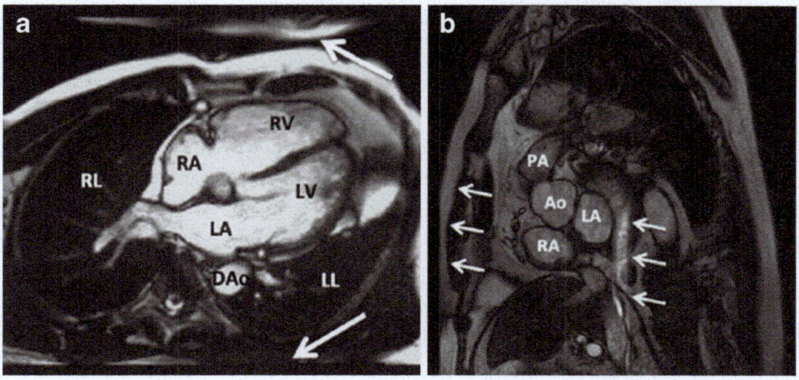

Fig. 14.5 Wrap-around artefact in panel A (see white arrow). When acceleration techniques are used to fasten image acquisition and the FOV is too small, anatomical parts not included in the FOV are wrapped into the middle of the image (panel **b**). From Neth Heart J (2014) 22:542–549. Open access

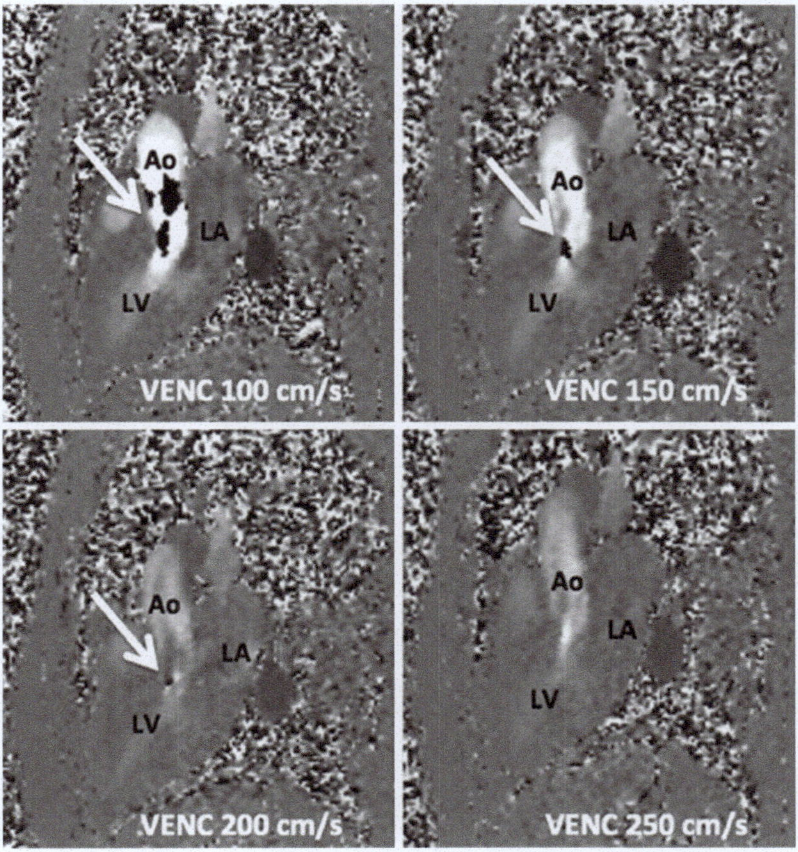

Fig. 14.6 Aliasing in a phase contrast image to evaluate a dynamic gradient in hypertrophic cardiomyopathy (HCM) in the LV outflow tract (LVOT). Increasing the selected values of VENC from 100 to 250 cm/s, the aliasing (black areas within the LVOT) is eliminated. Modified from Neth Heart J (2014) 22:542–549. Open access

14.5 Chemical-Shift Artefacts

Resonance frequency of water and fat differs by 210 Hz at 1.5 tesla; it is possible to have a misregistration between fat- and water-based tissues. There are two main types: (1) cine sequences and (2) still images. A typical example for cine imaging is signal cancellation in an apical thrombus (Fig. 14.7a). Another example can occur in still images, since fat and water have difference resonance frequencies, their reconstruction can occur in different space positions due to this chemical shift (Fig. 14.7b). The distance of separation will depend on the receiver bandwidth. For example, if the bandwidth was 105 Hz/pixel, then at 1.5 T their separation of 210 Hz would equate to 2 pixels on the reconstructed image. If the bandwidth were doubled to 210 Hz, then the separation would be halved to 1 pixel. Clearly the chemical-shift effect is reduced by increasing the bandwidth. This advantage, however, has to be balanced against the loss of signal to noise ratio (SNR).

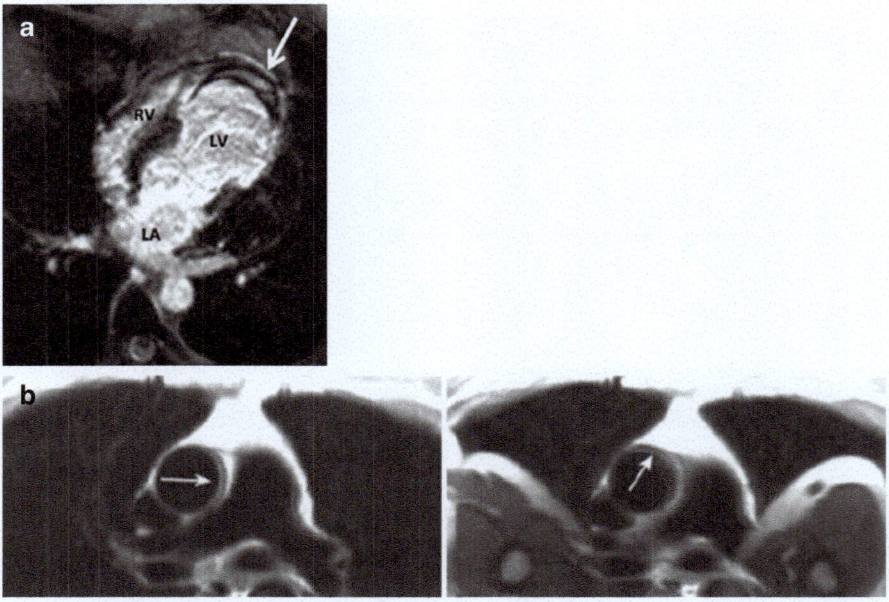

Fig. 14.7 (**a**) Chemical-shift artefact with hypointense signal from the core of an apical thrombus (see white arrow); modified from Neth Heart J (2014) 22:542–549. Open access. (**b**) Chemical-shift artefact in black-blood T1w still images at the interface blood/arterial wall (see white arrows). This artefact may simulate aortic dissection and should be appropriately interpreted to avoid misdiagnosis. Modified from Ferreira et al. Journal of Cardiovascular Magnetic Resonance 2013, 15:41. Open access

14.6 Magnetic Field Inhomogeneity Artefacts

Implanted medical devices can affect the homogeneity of main magnetic field and be responsible of loss of signals and part of the diagnostic images (Fig. 14.8). Cine sequences are especially affected by this type of artefact.

Another potential source of distortion of the main magnetic field can be caused by external radio frequencies (e.g. magnetic room door open, damage of the Faraday cab isolating the main magnetic room from external interferences). Such interferences may produce a typical artefact named "zipper artefact" since it shows a number of parallel lines mimicking a zipper.

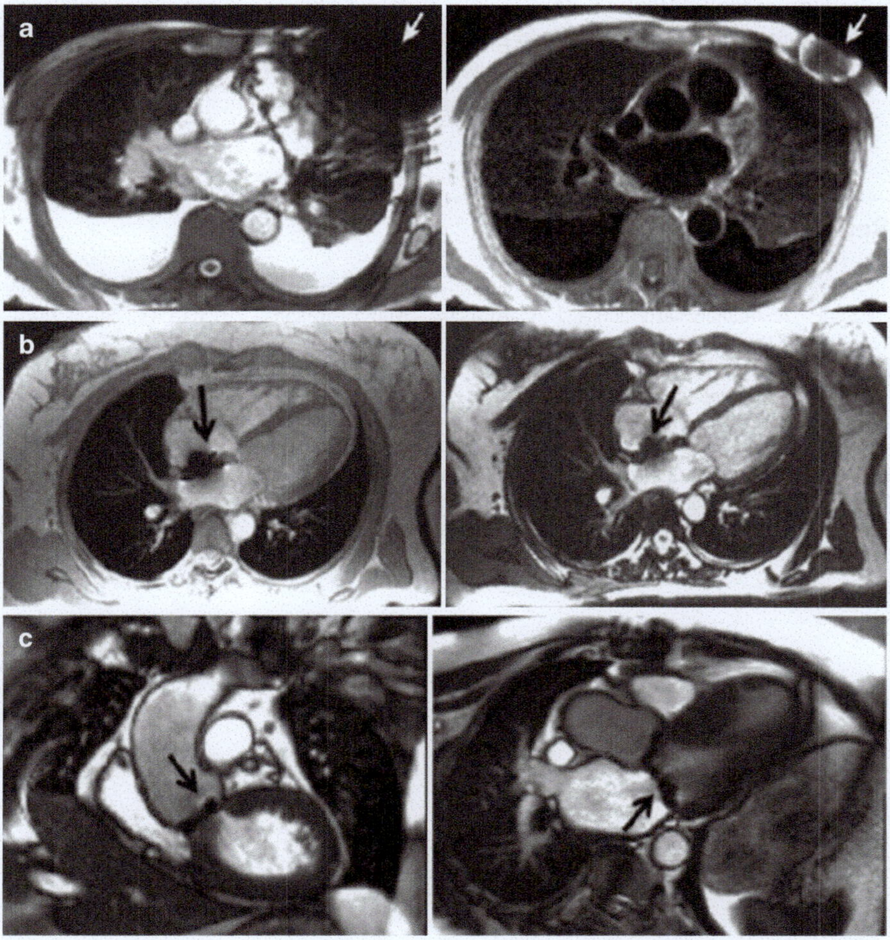

Fig. 14.8 Inhomogeneities of the main magnetic field with signal losses by different implanted devices: (**a**) loop recorder, (**b**) septal occluder and (**c**) heart valves. Modified from Ferreira et al. Journal of Cardiovascular Magnetic Resonance 2013, 15:41. Open access

14.7 Key Points

- CMR is prone to artefacts since it is depicting a moving organ because of cardiac contractions, breathing and blood flows but also because of different tissue characteristics (fat, muscle, blood) and possible presence of devices.
- An artefact is a finding on MR images that is not real, but it is produced incidentally by the use of specific techniques and sequences.
- An artefact may affect the quality of the images and reduce diagnostic capabilities.
- Knowledge of artefacts that are generated during the acquisition process is important to make corrections and reduce the negative impact of artefacts on the quality of the CMR exam.
- Main artefacts in CMR imaging include (1) movement artefacts (breathing, cardiac, flow-related), (2) truncation artefacts (Gibbs ringing), (3) aliasing artefacts, (4) chemical-shift artefacts and (5) magnetic field inhomogeneity artefacts.

References

1. Ferreira PF, Gatehouse PD, Mohiaddin RH, Firmin DN. Cardiovascular magnetic resonance artefacts. J Cardiovasc Magn Reson. 2013;15:41. https://doi.org/10.1186/1532-429X-15-41.
2. van der Graaf AW, Bhagirath P, Ghoerbien S, Götte MJ. Cardiac magnetic resonance imaging: artefacts for clinicians. Neth Hear J. 2014;22(12):542–9.
3. Ridgway JP. Cardiovascular magnetic resonance physics for clinicians: part I. J Cardiovasc Magn Reson. 2010;12:71.
4. Biglands JD, Radjenovic A, Ridgway JP. Cardiovascular magnetic resonance physics for clinicians: Part II. J Cardiovasc Magn Reson. 2012;14:66.

Incidental Findings

15

Contents

15.1 Introduction

In CMR the initial evaluation is conducted by low-resolution sequences to localize the heart and acquire basic views of the heart. Incidentally several additional anatomical parts are depicted both in the neck, thorax and upper abdomen making possible the detection of incidental findings related to extracardiac organs [1]. In a recent systematic review of 12 studies conducted on >7000 patients, extracardiac findings have been detected in 35% of cases, and such findings were major in 12% of cases. In about 1% of cases, such findings had an impact on subsequent management [2]. The evaluation of such findings will probably increase in the future since more CMR exams will be performed in a progressively older population with more comorbidities [3].

Such findings may be important for different reasons: (1) clinical management (diagnosis of cardiac and/or extracardiac involvement of a disease), (2) possibility to start new therapies and (3) ethical and medico-legal issues. The report of CMR is variable; usually a technician performs the CMR exam under the supervision of a physician trained in CMR (radiologist and/or cardiologist). In this setting,

M. Imazio et al., *Learning Cardiac Magnetic Resonance*,
https://doi.org/10.1007/978-3-030-11608-8_15

Table 15.1 Main extrcardiac findings according to their localization

1. Neck
(a) Thyroid nodules
(b) Cervical adenopathy
2. Thorax
(a) Lung (airway disease, mass)
(b) Pleura (effusion, neoplasm)
(c) Mediastinum (oesophagus diseases: e.g. hernia, mass, dilatation/thickening, mediastinal masses and cysts and adenopathies)
(d) Chest wall and bones (breast, axilla, fractures, neoplasm, infections)
3. Upper abdomen
(a) Liver (cyst, hemangioma, mass, parenchymal diseases) and biliary tract (gallstones, cholecystitis)
(b) Kidney (cyst, mass, hydronephrosis, parenchymal disease)
(c) Adrenal mass
(d) Spleen
(e) Ascites

radiological opinion is important. Low-resolution images usually do not allow a comprehensive evaluation of the extracardiac finding, and additional investigations may be needed. Main extracardiac findings are reported in Table 15.1 and may be detected in the neck, mediastinum, thorax, upper abdomen, chest wall and bones. A detailed description of each extracardiac finding is beyond the purpose of the present text. This introductory appendix will deal with general aspects of main extracardiac findings. Additional readings are reported in the reference list [1–6].

15.2 Neck

Main extracardiac findings in the neck are related to the thyroid and cervical adenopathies.

Localizer images and cross-sectional anatomical sequences, e.g. axial black-blood imaging, usually demonstrate a part of the cervical region and upper mediastinum.

More common extracardiac findings of the thyroid gland are represented by goitre (most common in postmenopausal women) or thyroid nodules. Retrosternal extension of a goitre and compressive effects on trachea (trachea deviation) can be shown by CMR (Fig. 15.1). Low-resolution images do not allow to identify benign and malignant nature of nodules. According to the American College of Radiology, a thyroid nodule that has been detected as incidental finding on CMR should undergo further evaluation by ultrasonography if >1 cm in patients with <35 years or >1.5 cm in patients with >35 years in the absence of signs of local invasion and associated adenopathies [4].

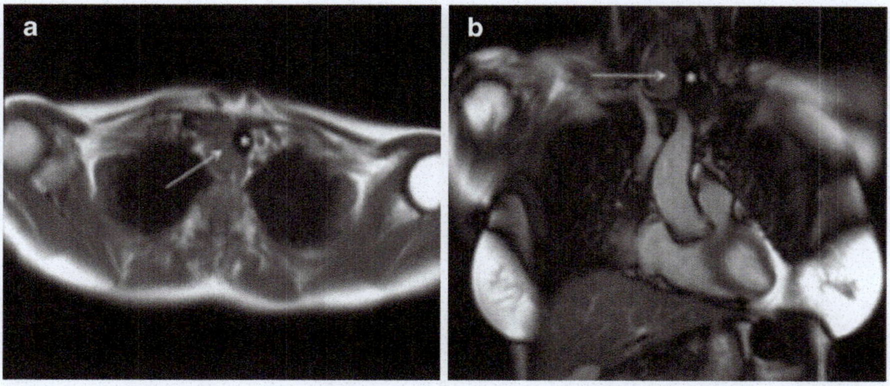

Fig. 15.1 Thyroid goitre with tracheal deviation (see white arrows). From Rodrigues et al. Journal of Cardiovascular Magnetic Resonance (2016) 18:26. Open access

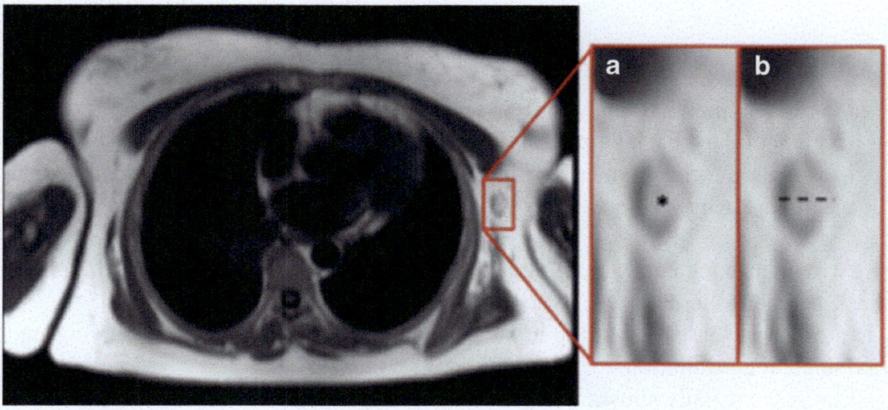

Fig. 15.2 Normal aspect of an axillary lymphonode: fatty hilum with a short axis <10 mm. From Rodrigues et al. Journal of Cardiovascular Magnetic Resonance (2016) 18:26. Open access

15.3 Mediastinum and Lungs

The main diseases of the mediastinum and lungs that can be detected on CMR include:

1. *Adenopathies* (normal lymphonodes have a characteristic morphology with a fatty hilum; the short-axis diameter should be quoted and not the maximum dimension of the node. A normal dimension is less than 10 mm. Nevertheless low-resolution imaging and slice thickness >5 mm preclude an adequate assessment of the size of mediastinal lymphonodes) (Fig. 15.2).

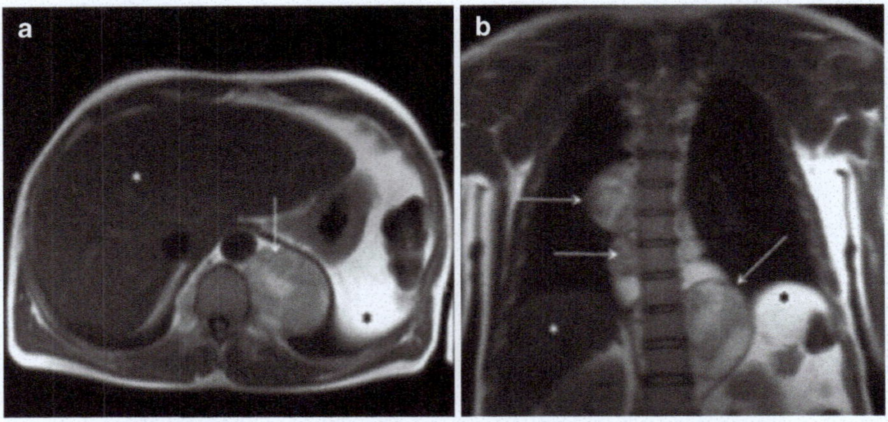

Fig. 15.3 Extramedullary haematopoiesis in a patient with thalassaemia. From Rodrigues et al. Journal of Cardiovascular Magnetic Resonance (2016) 18:26. Open access

2. Thymic remnants.
3. Masses (thymoma, lymphoma and teratoma).
4. Extramedullary haematopoiesis is seen more frequently in centres where T2* MRI is used for assessment of myocardial and hepatic iron loading in, for example, thalassaemia patients (Fig. 15.3).

A frequent incidental finding that may mimic an inferior posterior mediastinal mass is a hiatus hernia.

In all these cases, it is important the comparison with previous imaging and radiological consultation.

Lungs are usually shown in axial low-resolution scans. Assessment of the lung parenchyma is often limited by a combination of respiratory motion artefact, low proton density of the aerated lung parenchyma and the presence of susceptibility artefact occurring at air-tissue interfaces. Nevertheless pulmonary abnormalities can be detected in about 20% of patients. A common normal variant is the azygous lobe fissure that is found in 1–2% of population. It occurs as the displaced azygous vein makes a deep invagination into the apical segment of the right upper lobe; since it lacks its own bronchus, it is not a true anatomical accessory lobe (Fig. 15.4).

Most common pulmonary abnormalities are pulmonary opacities: they are named nodules if <3 cm and masses if greater than 3 cm (Fig. 15.5). Nodule size is the main predictor of malignancy. The presence of irregular margins and local invasion are also suggestive of malignancy.

One of the more common thoracic extracardiac findings is represented by pleural effusion that has a low intensity on T1-weighted and high intensity on T2-weighted images (watery content).

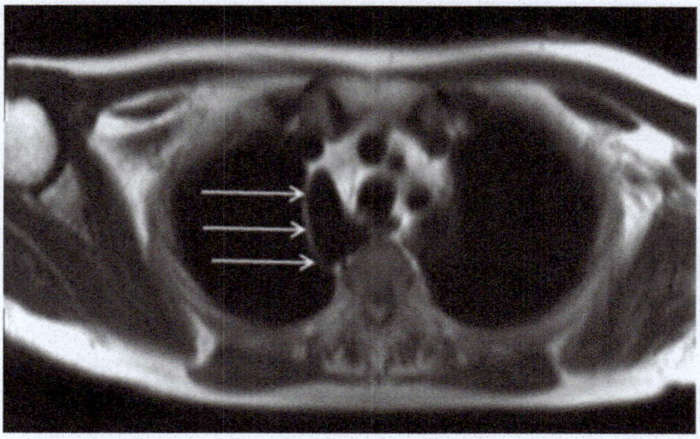

Fig. 15.4 Azygous lobe fissure (see white arrows). From Rodrigues et al. Journal of Cardiovascular Magnetic Resonance (2016) 18:26. Open access

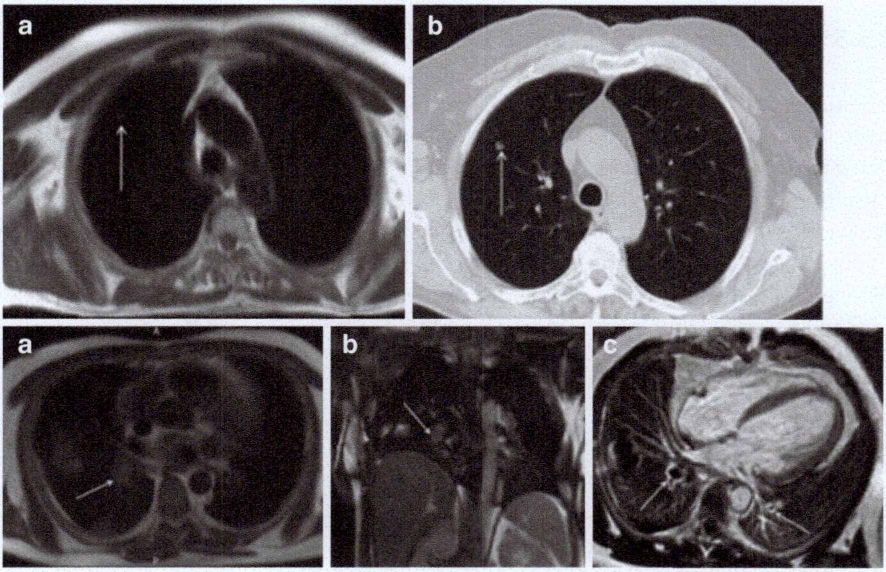

Fig. 15.5 Incidental finding of a lung nodule (upper panel **a**) confirmed by CT (upper panel **b**). A case of pulmonary embolism is reported in lower panels (**a–c**) (see white arrows). From Rodrigues et al. Journal of Cardiovascular Magnetic Resonance (2016) 18:26. Open access

15.4 Breast

Incidental breast lesions can be detected in up to 2.5% of CMR studies (Fig. 15.6). Breast undergoes fibro-fatty replacement with aging, and these changes may be asymmetrical and a focus of persistent glandular tissue may mimic a breast lesion. The finding of a breast lesion should trigger a referral for additional evaluation since low-resolution images are not diagnostic. A special care should be taken to evaluate signs of local invasion and adenopathies, especially if associated with a previous history of breast cancer or radiotherapy.

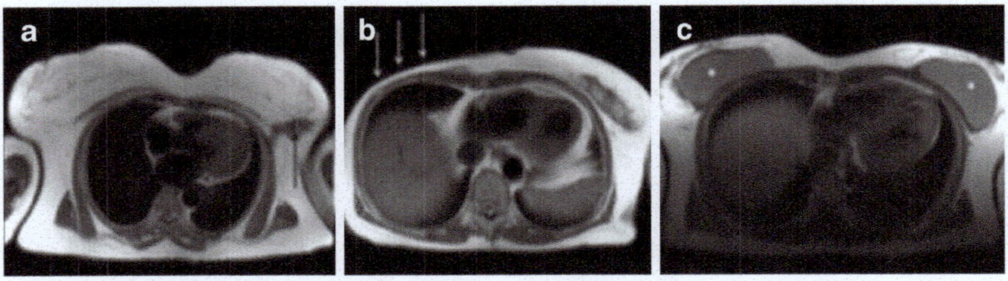

Fig. 15.6 Axial black-blood imaging showing a breast mass (see panel **a** with black arrow), previous right-sided mastectomy (see panel **b**) and bilateral breast prostheses (see panel **c**). From Rodrigues et al. Journal of Cardiovascular Magnetic Resonance (2016) 18:26. Open access

15.5 Liver, Biliary Tract and Other Abdominal Findings

The more common incidental findings are represented by renal cysts. Also for the liver, hepatic cysts are the most common incidental findings. Hepatic cysts have generally high signal return from T2-weighted imaging. The main issue is when to raise the suspicion of a malignant lesion of the liver: a malignant lesion (e.g. liver metastases) is variable in their T1 and T2 signal intensities but usually result in hypo- to isointense signal on T1-weighted images and iso- to hyperintense signal on T2-weighted images; often its margin are irregular (Fig. 15.7). Liver metastases tend to lose signal with increasing T2 weighting, whereas liver cysts and hemangiomas remain bright. The subsequent first level referral is for abdominal ultrasonography.

Gallbladder may display gallstones in 10–15% of patients. Calcific gallstones have low signal, while cholesterol stones have a high signal on T1-weighted imaging. Cholecystitis is characterized by wall thickening and pericholecystic fluid, with possible biliary tree dilatation, raising the possibility of choledocholithiasis. However such findings are unusual if gallstone disease is detected incidentally at CMR.

As mentioned, more common incidental findings at the level of kidneys (normal long axis is 10–12 cm) are represented by renal cysts. Most of these lesions will be simple benign cysts of no clinical relevance. However, a proportion of cystic renal lesions have malignant potential. Completely simple cysts, with a diameter <3 cm, have virtually no malignant potential, but complex cysts with multiple septations and nodules as well as part-solid, part-cystic components are highly concerning for malignancy. If available, the lack of cyst enhancement is a reassuring feature (Fig. 15.8).

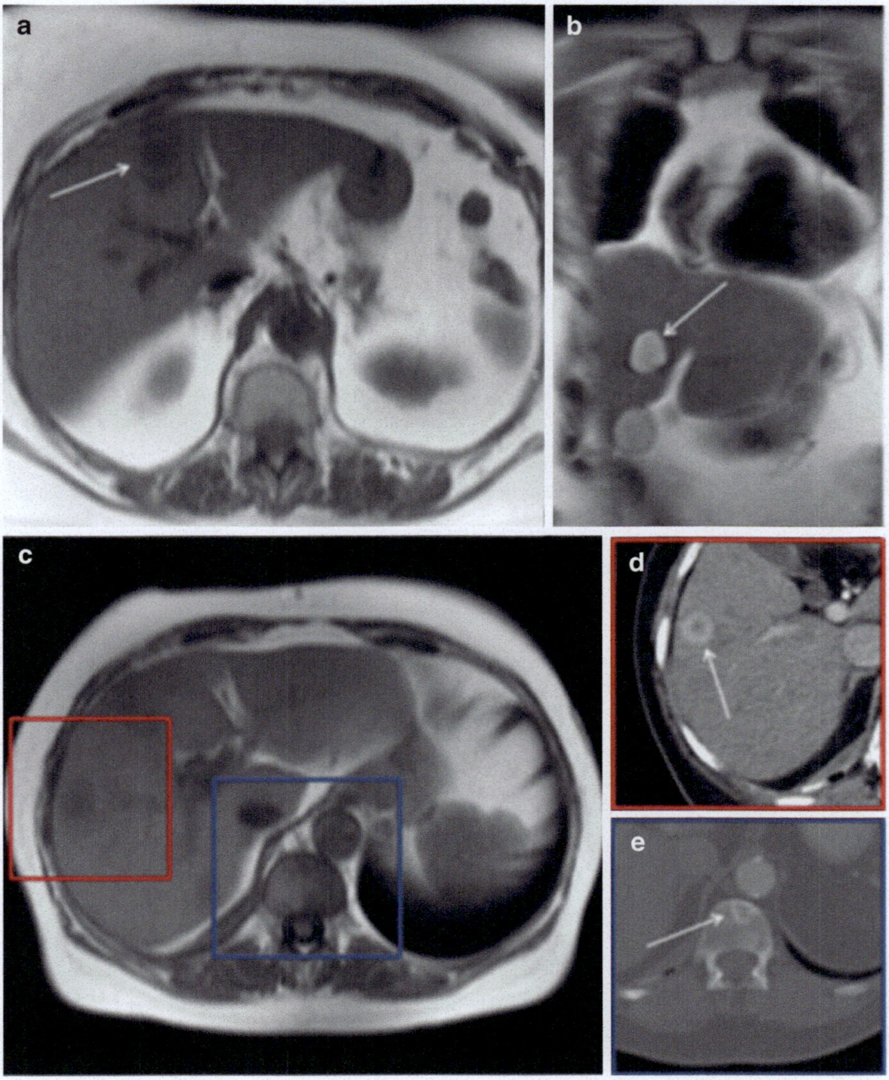

Fig. 15.7 Liver cystic lesions (**a** and **b**). Cystic lesion with not well-defined borders, low signal intensity (panel **c**) that is better characterized as secondary lesion with also a vertebral lesion on CT (panels **d** and **e**). From Rodrigues et al. Journal of Cardiovascular Magnetic Resonance (2016) 18:26. Open access

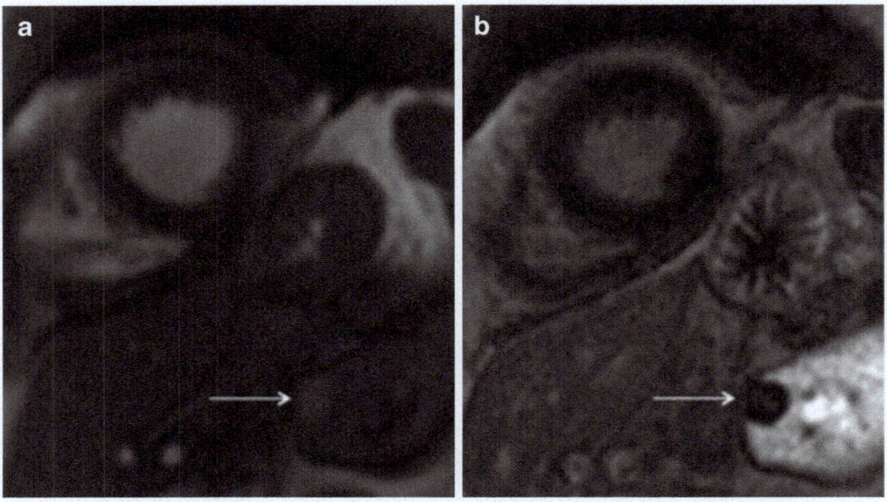

Fig. 15.8 Benign renal cyst with a high signal on cine imaging (panel **a**) and no cystic uptake of contrast agent (panel **b**). From Rodrigues et al. Journal of Cardiovascular Magnetic Resonance (2016) 18:26. Open access

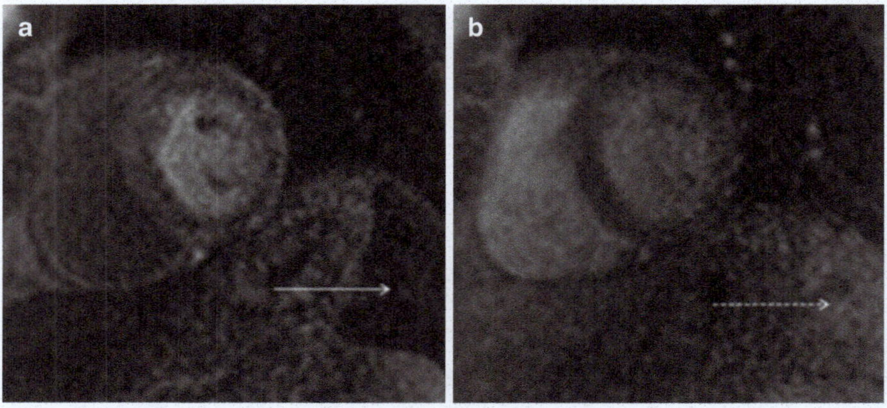

Fig. 15.9 Splenic switch-off after adenosine administration in a CMR stress test (panel **a**); at rest the spleen has regular uptake of contrast (panel **b**). From Rodrigues et al. Journal of Cardiovascular Magnetic Resonance (2016) 18:26. Open access

The normal spleen has a long axis of 11–12 cm. The most common pathological findings are represented by splenomegaly that should be correlated with the underlying disease. Under stress conditions (e.g. exercise or pharmacological stimulation), the spleen undergoes vasoconstriction ("splenic switch-off"). This finding can be used to assess good stimulation by adenosine during a stress test (Fig. 15.9).

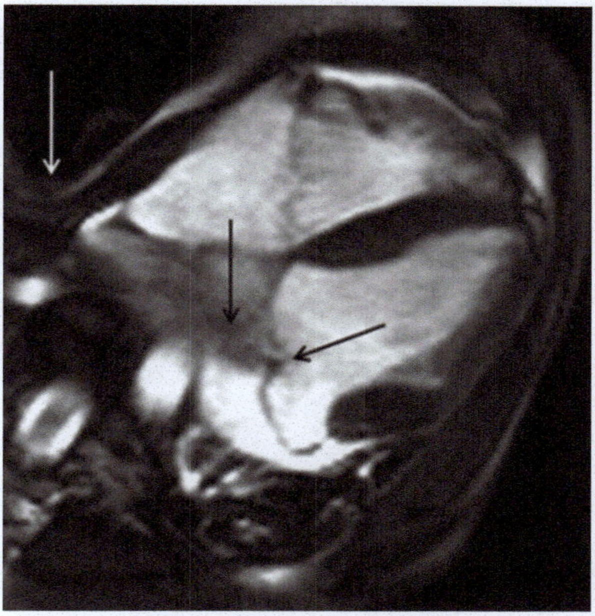

Fig. 15.10 Pectum excavatum (see white arrow) and mitral valve prolapse (black arrows) in a patient with Marfan syndrome. From Rodrigues et al. Journal of Cardiovascular Magnetic Resonance (2016) 18:26. Open access

15.6 Bones and Thoracic Rib Cage

One of the most common findings is represented by abnormalities of the chest wall such as pectus excavatum that can be associated with other structural abnormalities (e.g. mitral valve prolapse) and Marfan syndrome (Fig. 15.10).

In addition, lesions of the thoracic vertebral bodies can be found on CMR low-resolution images. The most common lesion is hemangioma (Fig. 15.11) that should be considered also in the differential diagnosis with metastases (see Table 15.2 for differential diagnosis according to features on T1- and T2-weighted images).

15.7 Key Points

- Low-resolution sequences used as localizers at the beginning of a CMR exam may allow to visualize incidental finding in the neck, thorax and upper abdomen.
- Such incidental findings are reported in 1/3 of patients and are major findings in 10% of cases with the potentiality to affect subsequent management of the patients in up to 1% of cases.
- The recognition of incidental findings is important from a clinical, ethical and medico-legal point of view.

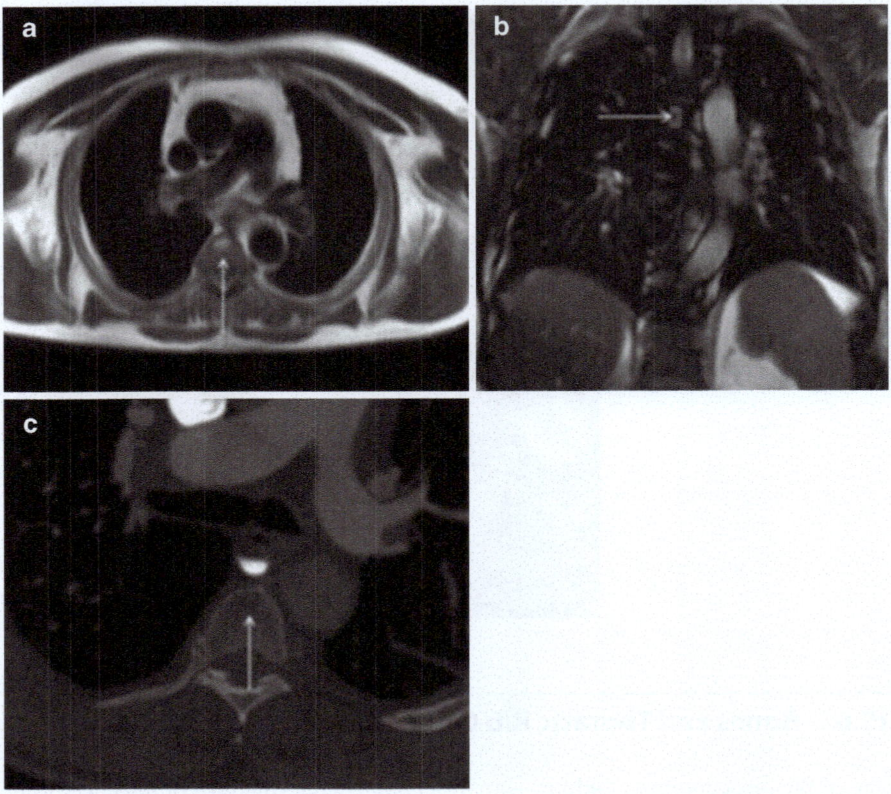

Fig. 15.11 Thoracic vertebral hemangioma as low intensity signal on low-resolution images (axial in panel **a** and coronal in panel **b**) with typical appearance with "polka dot sign" on CT imaging (panel **c**). From Rodrigues et al. Journal of Cardiovascular Magnetic Resonance (2016) 18:26. Open access

Table 15.2 Differential RM diagnosis of hemangioma vs. metastases (osteoblastic or osteolytic) according to RM sequences

Lesion	T1-weighted	T2-weighted
Hemangioma (=fat and vessels)	High signal (bright on T1w)	High signal
Osteoblastic (=osteogenic lesion)	Low signal	Low signal
Osteolytic (=lesion with bone reabsorption)	Low signal	Low signal

- The main extracardiac findings in the cervical zone are represented by goitre, thyroid nodules and cervical lymphoadenopathies.
- Breast lesion can be encountered and warrant additional evaluation by dedicated imaging since low-resolution images are not sufficient for the precise diagnosis.
- Incidental lung findings are reported in about 20% of scans and are especially nodules or masses, lymphoadenopathies and pleural effusion.
- Most common abdominal findings are renal and hepatic cysts.

- Most common bone lesions are thoracic vertebral hemangioma or metastases (either osteoblastic or osteolytic lesions) that can be initially assessed according to their aspect on T1- and T2-weighted imaging by MR.

References

1. Bruder O, Wagner A, Lombardi M, Schwitter J, van Rossum A, Pilz G, Nothnagelv D, Steen H, Petersen S, Nagel E, Prasad S, Schumm J, Greulich S, Cagnolo A, Monney P, Deluigi CC, Dill T, Frank H, Sabin G, Schneider S, Mahrholdt H. European Cardiovascular Magnetic Resonance (EuroCMR) registry—multi national results from 57 centers in 15 countries. J Cardiovasc Magn Reson. 2013;15:9.
2. Dunet V, Schwitter J, Meuli R, Beigelman-Aubry C. Incidental extracardiac findings on cardiac MR: systematic review and meta-analysis. J Magn Reson Imaging. 2016;43(4):929–39. https://doi.org/10.1002/jmri.25053.
3. Rodrigues JC, Lyen SM, Loughborough W, Amadu AM, Baritussio A, Dastidar AG, Manghat NE, Bucciarelli-Ducci C. Extra-cardiac findings in cardiovascular magnetic resonance: what the imaging cardiologist needs to know. J Cardiovasc Magn Reson. 2016;18(1):26.
4. Hoang JK, Langer JE, Middleton WD, Wu CC, Hammers LW, Cronan JJ, et al. Managing incidental thyroid nodules detected on imaging: white paper of the ACR Incidental Thyroid Findings Committee. J Am Coll Radiol Elsevier. 2015;12(2):143–50.
5. Gravina M, Stoppino LP, Casavecchia G, Moffa AP, Vinci R, Brunetti ND, Di Biase M, Macarini L. Incidental extracardiac findings and their characterization on cardiac MRI. Biomed Res Int. 2017;2017:2423546. https://doi.org/10.1155/2017/2423546.
6. Sohns JM, Menke J, Schwarz A, Bergau L, Kowallick JT, Schuster A, Konietschke F, Placzek M, Weiberg D, Nordlohne S, Schmuck S, Schulz S, Derlin T, Staab W. Incidental findings in cardiac magnetic resonance imaging: superiority of bSSFP over T1w-HASTE for extra-cardiac findings assessment. Int J Cardiovasc Imaging. 2017;33(10):1581–7. https://doi.org/10.1007/s10554-017-1145-8.

The manufacturer's authorised representative in the EU is Springer
Nature Customer Service Centre GmbH, Europaplatz 3, 69115 Heidelberg,
Germany. If you have any concerns regarding our products, please
contact ProductSafety@springernature.com

Printed and bound by CPI Group (UK) Ltd, Croydon, CR0 4YY
05/10/2026
02228129-0001